theclinics.com

IMMUNOLOGY AND ALLERGY CLINICS OF NORTH AMERICA

Novel Aspects of Native and Recombinant Allergens and their Therapeutic Implications

GUEST EDITOR
Sanjiv Sur, MD

CONSULTING EDITOR
Rafeul Alam, MD, PhD

February 2007 • Volume 27 • Number 1

SAUNDERS

An Imprint of Elsevier, Inc.
PHILADELPHIA LONDON TORONTO MONTREAL SYDNEY TOKYO

W.B. SAUNDERS COMPANY
A Division of Elsevier Inc.

Elsevier, Inc., 1600 John F. Kennedy Blvd., Suite 1800, Philadelphia, PA 19103-2899

http://www.theclinics.com

IMMUNOLOGY AND ALLERGY CLINICS OF NORTH AMERICA
February 2007
Editor: Carla Holloway

Volume 27, Number 1
ISSN 0889-8561
ISBN 1-4160-4325-X
978-1-4160-4325-6

Immunology and Allergy Clinics of North America (ISSN 0889-8561) is published quarterly by Elsevier Inc., 360 Park Avenue South, New York, NY 10010-1710. Months of issue are February, May, August, and November. Business and Editorial offices: 1600 John F. Kennedy Blvd., Suite 1800, Philadelphia, PA 19103-2899. Customer Service office: 6277 Sea Harbor Drive, Orlando, FL 32887-4800. Periodicals postage paid at New York, NY and additional mailing offices. Subscription prices are $193.00 per year for US individuals, $308.00 per year for US institutions, $94.00 per year for US students and residents, $237.00 per year for Canadian individuals, $127.00 for Canadian students and residents, $374.00 per year for Canadian institutions, $253.00 per year for international individuals, $374.00 per year for international institutions, $127.00 per year for international students. To receive student/resident rate, orders must be accompanied by name of affiliated institution, date of term, and the *signature* of program/residency coordinator on institution letterhead. Orders will be billed at individual rate until proof of status is received. Foreign air speed delivery is included in all *Clinics* subscription prices. All prices are subject to change without notice. POSTMASTER: Send address changes to *Immunology and Allergy Clinics of North America*, Elsevier Periodicals Customer Service, 6277 Sea Harbor Drive, Orlando, FL 32887-4800. **Customer Service: 1-800-654-2452 (US). From outside of the US, call 1-407-345-4000. E-mail: hhspcs@wbsaunders.com**.

Reprints. For copies of 100 or more, of articles in this publication, please contact the Commercial Reprints Department, Elsevier Inc., 360 Park Avenue South, New York, New York 10010-1710. Tel. (212) 633-3813 Fax: (212) 462-1935 e-mail: reprints@elsevier.com.

Immunology and Allergy Clinics of North America is covered in Index Medicus, Current Contents/Life Sciences, Science Citation Index, ISI/BIOMED, Chemical Abstracts, and EMBASE/Excerpta Medica.

Printed in the United States of America.

CONSULTING EDITOR

RAFEUL ALAM, MD, PhD, Veda and Chauncey Ritter Chair in Immunology; Professor and Director, Division of Allergy and Immunology, National Jewish Medical and Research Center; Co-Director, Immunology and Allergy, University of Colorado at Denver Health Sciences Center, Denver, Colorado

GUEST EDITOR

SANJIV SUR, MD, Professor of Medicine, Pediatrics, Microbiology, and Immunology, Division of Allergy, Pulmonary, Immunology, Critical Care and Sleep, Department of Internal Medicine, University of Texas Medical Branch, Galveston, Texas

CONTRIBUTORS

ATTILA BACSI, PhD, Assistant Professor, Institute of Immunology, University of Debrecen, Debrecen, Hungary

ISTVAN BOLDOGH, DMB, PhD, Professor of Microbiology and Immunology, Department of Microbiology and Immunology, University of Texas Medical Branch, Galveston, Texas

WERNER BRAUN, PhD, Professor and Vice-Chair, Sealy Center for Structural Biology and Molecular Biophysics, Department of Biochemistry and Molecular Biology, University of Texas Medical Branch, Galveston, Texas

RETO CRAMERI, PhD, Head, Division of Molecular Allergology, Swiss Institute of Allergy and Asthma Research (SIAF), Davos, Switzerland; Associate Professor of Immunology, Department of Molecular Biology, University of Salzburg, Salzburg, Austria

NILESH G. DHARAJIYA, MD, Scientist, Biomolecular Resource Facility, NHLBI Proteomics Center, Department of Biochemistry and Molecular Biology, University of Texas Medical Branch, Galveston, Texas

OLIVER DISSERTORI, BSc, Department of Molecular Biology, Division of Genomics, University of Salzburg, Salzburg, Austria

FATIMA FERREIRA, PhD, Associate Professor, Department of Molecular Biology, Christian Doppler Laboratory for Allergy Diagnostic and Therapy, University of Salzburg, Salzburg, Austria

OVIDIU IVANCIUC, PhD, Sealy Center for Structural Biology and Molecular Biophysics, Department of Biochemistry and Molecular Biology, University of Texas Medical Branch, Galveston, Texas

CHRISTOPHER KEPLEY, PhD, Division of Rheumatology, Allergy, and Immunology, Department of Internal Medicine, Virginia Commonwealth University Health System, Richmond, Virginia

PETER LACKNER, PhD, Associate Professor, Department of Molecular Biology, Division of Genomics, University of Salzburg, Salzburg, Austria

ANNA NOWACK-WEGRZYN, MD, Assistant Professor of Pediatrics, Jaffe Food Allergy Institute, Division of Allergy and Immunology, Department of Pediatrics, Mount Sinai School of Medicine, New York, New York

STEVEN A. PORCELLI, MD, Professor, Department of Microbiology and Immunology; and Department of Internal Medicine, Albert Einstein College of Medicine, Bronx, New York

CLAUDIO RHYNER, PhD, Senior Scientist, Division of Molecular Allergology, Swiss Institute of Allergy and Asthma Research (SIAF), Davos, Switzerland

ANDREW SAXON, MD, The Hart and Louise Lyon Laboratory, Division of Clinical Immunology/Allergy, Department of Medicine, UCLA School of Medicine, Los Angeles, California

CATHERINE H. SCHEIN, PhD, Associate Professor, Sealy Center for Structural Biology and Molecular Biophysics, Department of Biochemistry and Molecular Biology; and Department of Microbiology and Immunology, University of Texas Medical Branch, Galveston, Texas

FABRIZIO SPINOZZI, MD, Associate Professor of Medicine, Experimental Immunology and Allergy, Department of Clinical and Experimental Medicine, University of Perugia, Perugia, Italy

SANJIV SUR, MD, Professor of Medicine, Pediatrics, Microbiology, and Immunology, Division of Allergy, Pulmonary, Immunology, Critical Care and Sleep, Department of Internal Medicine, University of Texas Medical Branch, Galveston, Texas

FUMO TAKAIWA, PhD, Chief of Research Center, Transgenic Crop Research and Development Center, National Institute of Agrobiological Sciences, Tsukuba Ibaraki, Japan

TETSUYA TERADA, MD, PhD, The Hart and Louis Lyon Laboratory, Division of Clinical Immunology/Allergy, Department of Medicine, UCLA School of Medicine, Los Angeles, California; Department of Otorhinolaryngology, Osaka Medical College, Takatsuki, Osaka, Japan

NICOLE WOPFNER, PhD, Research Assistant, Department of Molecular Biology, Christian Doppler Laboratory for Allergy Diagnostic and Therapy, University of Salzburg, Salzburg, Austria

KE ZHANG, MD, PhD, The Hart and Louise Lyon Laboratory, Division of Clinical Immunology/Allergy, Department of Medicine, UCLA School of Medicine, Los Angeles, California

DAOCHENG ZHU, PhD, Division of Allergy/Immunology, Department of Medicine, Northwestern University, Chicago, Illinois

CONTENTS

Foreword xiii
Rafeul Alam

Preface xv
Sanjiv Sur

Bioinformatics Approaches to Classifying Allergens and Predicting Cross-Reactivity 1
Catherine H. Schein, Ovidiu Ivanciuc, and Werner Braun

Allergenic proteins from very different environmental sources have similar sequences and structures. This fact may account for multiple allergen syndromes, whereby a myriad of diverse plants and foods may induce a similar IgE-based reaction in certain patients. Identifying the common triggering protein in these sources, in silico, can aid designing individualized therapy for allergen sufferers. This article provides an overview of databases on allergenic proteins, and ways to identify common proteins that may be the cause of multiple allergy syndromes. The major emphasis is on the relational Structural Database of Allergenic Proteins (SDAP [http://fermi.utmb.edu/SDAP/]), which includes cross-referenced data on the sequence, structure, and IgE epitopes of over 800 allergenic proteins, coupled with specially developed bioinformatics tools to group all allergens and identify discrete areas that may account for cross-reactivity. SDAP is freely available on the Web to clinicians and patients.

Calcium-Binding Proteins and their Role in Allergic Diseases 29
Nicole Wopfner, Oliver Dissertori, Fatima Ferreira, and Peter Lackner

Calcium-binding proteins (CBPs) are ubiquitous pollen allergens and important food allergens in fish and amphibians.

Calcium-binding allergens containing two EF-hands (polcalcins) have been detected and characterized in pollen from trees, grasses, and weeds. Timothy grass Phl p 7 is the most cross-reactive allergen among polcalcins. Although there is cross-reactivity described within the subfamilies of calcium-binding allergens, there are no strong indications for IgE cross-reactivity between CBPs from plants, fish, and humans. Therefore, Phl p 7 could be used as marker to identify multiple pollen-sensitized patients, whereas cod Gad c 1 or carp Cyp c 1 could be selected for the diagnosis of fish allergy. Hom s 4, a calcium-binding autoantigen, might be an interesting candidate to monitor chronic skin inflammation in atopic and nonatopic individuals. Diagnostic tests containing these molecules could allow the identification of most patients sensitized to calcium-binding allergens/antigens. In general, IgE recognition of calcium-binding allergens is influenced by binding or release of calcium ions. This knowledge could be used to engineer hypoallergenic CBPs for specific immunotherapy.

Pollen NAD(P)H Oxidases and their Contribution to Allergic Inflammation **45**

Nilesh G. Dharajiya, Attila Bacsi, Istvan Boldogh, and Sanjiv Sur

This article provides an overview of NADPH oxidase and its role in allergic inflammation. A background and historical perspectives of NADPH oxidase are first provided, followed by a detailed overview of mammalian NADPH oxidase subunits and their functional organization. Plant NADPH oxidase, the authors' discovery of NADPH oxidase in pollens, and their contribution to allergic inflammation are then discussed, concluding with a discussion of future directions and outstanding questions that require attention.

Impact of Native, Recombinant, and Cross-Reactive Allergens on Humoral and T-Cell—Mediated Immune Responses **65**

Reto Crameri and Claudio Rhyner

Many native allergens have been purified to homogeneity from natural sources, and whole arrays of recombinant and cross-reactive allergens have been produced in large amounts as biologically active molecules. These allergens offer potent research tools to investigate humoral and T cell—mediated immune responses to allergens in healthy and allergic individuals, providing methods for verifying the responses in a reproducible and dose-dependent manner. Dissecting the immune responses to allergens at cellular and molecular levels provides models for studying the different aspects of T-cell activation and the development of immunologic memory and effector functions. A deep understanding of these mechanisms will fundamentally change the current practice of allergy diagnosis, treatment, and prevention.

Recognition of Lipids from Pollens by CD1-Restricted T Cells 79
Fabrizio Spinozzi and Steven A. Porcelli

Allergic rhinitis and asthma should be considered as organ-specific inflammatory diseases in which the genetic background has determined a local overproduction of Th2-type cytokines and an overexpansion of particular APCs and T cells. Among the latter, a potential pathogenetic role could be assumed for natural killer T cells, expressing both invariant ($V\alpha24/V\beta11$) and classic $\alpha\beta$ or $\gamma\delta$ T-cell receptors. Recent studies support this notion and also suggest that surface pollen substances of nonprotein structure, such as lipid components recognized by CD1, could be viewed as one of the foreign materials against which the immune system of the allergic subject can mount a local inflammatory response.

Chimeric Human Fcγ—Allergen Fusion Proteins in the Prevention of Allergy 93
Ke Zhang, Daocheng Zhu, Christopher Kepley, Tetsuya Terada, and Andrew Saxon

Allergic responses are strongly associated with Th2-type immune responses, and modulation of the skewed Th2 response toward a more balanced response is the major goal of allergen immunotherapy (IT) in allergic disorders. To achieve this goal, several approaches have been tested. The authors previously showed that a human immunoglobulin (Ig) Fcγ—Fcε fusion protein (GE2) that directly cross-links FcεRI and FcγRIIb on human mast cells and basophils was able to inhibit degranulation, and they reasoned that human gamma—allergen fusion protein would achieve a similar inhibitory effect in an allergen-specific fashion while preserving the immunogenicity of the allergen component. Therefore, the authors constructed and developed a human—cat chimeric fusion protein composed of the human Fcγ1 and the cat allergen Fel d1 (*Felis domesticus*) for cat allergen—specific IT. This article summarizes the therapeutic features and potential of this novel fusion protein for allergic IT.

New Perspectives for Use of Native and Engineered Recombinant Food Proteins in Treatment of Food Allergy 105
Anna Nowak-Wegrzyn

Food allergy has emerged as an important target for research on curative treatment and prevention, with most efforts focusing on peanut, cow's milk, and egg allergy. This article reviews the recent developments in the potential treatments for IgE-mediated food allergy using native and engineered recombinant food proteins.

A Rice-Based Edible Vaccine Expressing Multiple T-Cell Epitopes to Induce Oral Tolerance and Inhibit Allergy **129**
Fumio Takaiwa

Plant pollens are the most common cause of seasonal allergic disease. The number of patients undergoing treatment for allergies to the pollen of Japanese cedar (major antigens, Cry j 1 and Cry j 2) has increased steadily each year. A rice seed—based edible vaccine has been shown to be effective for treating Japanese cedar pollinosis. Rice seeds containing the major T-cell epitopes derived from cedar pollen allergens were orally administrated to mice before systemic challenge with total pollen protein. Mucosal immune tolerance leading to a reduction of allergen-specific IgE, T-cell proliferative reactions, and histamine were induced, resulting in suppression of allergy-specific symptoms such as sneezing. Oral seed-based peptide immunotherapy offers a safe, simple, and cost-effective alternative to conventional allergen-specific immunotherapy using crude allergen extracts for treating allergic disease. A human version of rice seed—based edible vaccine containing seven T-cell epitopes from the Cry j 1 and Cry j 2 allergens was recently developed and is undergoing safety assessments.

Index **141**

FORTHCOMING ISSUES

May 2007

Anaphylaxis
Phil Lieberman, MD, *Guest Editor*

August 2007

Hypereosinophilic Syndrome: Pathogenesis and Management
Amy Klion, MD, *Guest Editor*

November 2007

Biomarkers in Allergy and Asthma
Rohit Katial, MD, FAAAAI, FACP, *Guest Editor*

RECENT ISSUES

November 2006

Angioedema
Bruce L. Zuraw, MD, *Guest Editor*

August 2006

Mast Cells and Mastocytosis
Cem Akin, MD, PhD, *Guest Editor*

May 2006

Allergen-Specific Immunotherapy
Cezmi Akdis, MD, *Guest Editor*

ELSEVIER
SAUNDERS

Immunol Allergy Clin N Am
27 (2007) xiii–xiv

IMMUNOLOGY
AND ALLERGY
CLINICS
OF NORTH AMERICA

Foreword

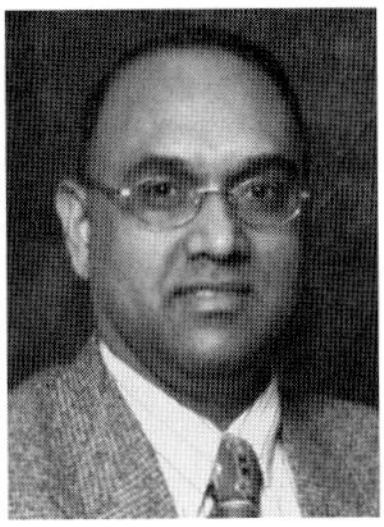

Rafeul Alam, MD, PhD
Consulting Editor

Allergens are, by definition, antigens that cause allergies. This definition points to an important difference between an antigen and an allergen, and we have yet to fully understand this difference. An understanding of this difference is important for several reasons. It is likely to provide a clue to the fact that allergens preferentially induce a Th2 immune response. The antigenic structure/sequence alone does not explain this bias for the Th2 response. It is likely that a pattern (eg, an allergen-associated molecular pattern) recognition mechanism is involved. Pattern recognition is the domain of the innate immune system and is mediated via toll-like receptors and non-TLR mechanisms. It is important to note that only a small fraction of the population is affected by allergies. Therefore, the host genetic background must be critically important. This issue of the *Immunology and Allergy Clinics of North America* addresses a few aspects of this important matter.

The study of allergen structure through the bioinformatic approach could not only facilitate the classification but also predict their function and immune response. Calcium-binding proteins are an example of this approach. They represent a structural pattern that is common to many allergens. The first two articles in this issue deal with these important structural aspects. For many years we have known that proteases play an important role in the allergenicity of dust mites and fungal antigens. Pollen-associated NADPH oxidase has now been identified as another component of allergens that is important for a robust allergic response. Interference with the NADPH oxidase prevents the development of allergy in the animal model.

doi:10.1016/j.iac.2007.01.001 *immunology.theclinics.com*

Allergen-associated lipids could constitute a molecular pattern for a biased immune response. The recognition of pollen-derived lipids by the non-polymorphic CD1 transmembrane protein is an exciting development, the relevance of which is discussed in the fifth article in this issue.

The second half of the issue is dedicated to novel interventions employing modified allergens. One approach is to eliminate the IgE-binding component and create linear fusion proteins of T cell epitopes. This genetically modified allergen vaccine is less likely to have serious side effects when compared with immunotherapy with conventional allergens. Another approach exploits mucosal tolerance to orally fed rice or killed bacteria that express recombinant allergens or their T cell epitopes. This "Trojan horse" approach has shown promise in the model of mountain cedar allergy and peanut allergy. A third approach takes advantage of the inhibitory signaling mechanism of FcRγII. The investigators have generated a fusion protein of the cat allergen and IgG—which, when it binds to mast cell–associated IgE, delivers an inhibitory signal through the IgG receptor. As a result, mast cell activation is blocked, and the allergic reaction is aborted. These clever approaches await clinical trials for their efficacy; nonetheless, they bring cutting edge molecular biology techniques to the bedside.

Rafeul Alam, MD, PhD
Division of Allergy and Immunology
National Jewish Medical and Research Center
University of Colorado Health Sciences Center
1400 Jackson Street
Denver, CO 80206, USA

E-mail address: alamr@njc.org

ELSEVIER
SAUNDERS

Immunol Allergy Clin N Am
27 (2007) xv–xviii

IMMUNOLOGY
AND ALLERGY
CLINICS
OF NORTH AMERICA

Preface

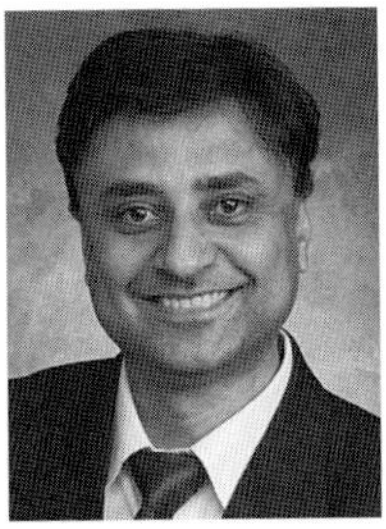

Sanjiv Sur, MD
Guest Editor

The mechanism of allergic inflammation has been studied extensively. However, considerably less is known about the properties of foods and inhaled substances in our environment that give them the ability to induce allergic symptoms. Scientists have been trying to understand the mechanisms underlying this fundamental question for decades. Over the years, investigators have identified many proteins in pollens, molds, animals and foods that bind IgE. As the field progressed, novel aspects of allergens other than their ability to bind IgE were discovered. Some of the most exciting developments in this field have occurred in the past decade, so I was delighted when the *Immunology and Allergy Clinics of North America* decided to dedicate an issue to the emerging field of "Novel Aspects of Native and Recombinant Allergens and their Therapeutic Implications."

I started thinking about how one could compile an intriguing and cohesive issue on this topic. The more I thought about it, the more I felt that it was fundamentally important to align with the current prevailing ideas of the scientific community, namely a "translational approach" similar to the NIH roadmap that begins with molecular and theoretical concepts and later examines information relevant to the clinician. Consequently, this issue has three broad groups of articles that together provide a "translational backbone."

The first set of articles relates to allergen structure and unique properties. The first article, by Schein and colleagues, begins with a bioinformatics

doi:10.1016/j.iac.2007.01.002
immunology.theclinics.com

approach to allergens and describes various Web sites that list known allergens, such as www.allergen.org and www.allergome.org. They then make a strong case for using one of them, the Structural Database of Allergenic Proteins (http://fermi.utmb.edu.SDAP), because it lists protein type, IgE epitope, experimental structures of allergens, and so forth. The article discusses grouping of allergen families based on structural similarities, such as proteases, EF-hands, and lipid transfer proteins that have extensive cross-reactivity. In the next article of this group, Wopfner and colleagues discuss in detail calcium-binding proteins that have calcium-binding domains termed EF-hands. Parvalbumin is a fish-derived allergen, and it was the first calcium-binding protein to be described about 30 years ago. Today the allergome database lists 64 calcium-binding allergens, 34 from pollen and 30 from animal sources. The authors note that IgE recognition of calcium-binding proteins is dependent on conformational changes induced by binding or release of calcium ions from these proteins. They also note that there is extensive cross-reactivity within subfamilies of calcium-binding proteins, but not across families. In the third article of this group, Dharajiya and colleagues discuss their recent discovery of pollen NADPH oxidases and its role in allergic inflammation. They first discuss the structure and function of mammalian NADPH oxidase, then compare plant NADPH oxidase to their mammalian counterpart. In the end, they review publications that have demonstrated that pollen NADPH oxidases provide a signal independent of adaptive immunity that plays a vital role in initiating allergic airway inflammation.

The second set of articles carefully examines immune responses induced by allergens. Crameri and Rhyner calculate that there are approximately 10^4 molecules that can elicit allergic symptoms, and suggest that many are cross-reactive. They describe IgE-mediated autoreactivity as a unique form of cross-reactivity in which self antigens are cross-reactive with known allergenic proteins. As an example, they describe human manganese superoxide dismutase (MnSOD), which shares greater than 50% homology with *Aspergillus fumigatus*. IgE from patients allergic to *Aspergillus* MnSOD cross-reacts with recombinant human, *Drosophila* and *Aspergillus* MnSOD, indicating molecular mimicry as a likely mechanism of this phenomenon. In the next article, Spinozzi and Porcelli examine the role of lipids in pollens as an inducer of immune responses. This article is unique because most prior studies of pollens have examined the role of soluble proteins as inducers of immune responses. They make a strong case for the role of lipid molecules in pollen external layers interacting with CD1a and CD1d molecules in dendritic cells as a mechanism of pollen capture. They go on to discuss their data demonstrating a role of lipid CD1 interaction in T cell activation and proliferation. They finally discuss that the cytokine response induced by this interaction is Th2 dominant in many cases, thereby contributing to allergic inflammation and IgE secretion.

The third set of articles examines strategies that are likely to have a preventive role in allergic diseases. One strategy is to generate fusion proteins between allergen and an inhibitory signaling molecule, such as the one described by Zhang and colleagues. Their group generated a fusion protein of Fel d 1, the major cat allergen, and FcgRIIb, an inhibitory signaling receptor that binds immunoglobulins. They discuss how this fusion protein blocks passive cutaneous anaphylaxis and allergic airway inflammation in mice, and prevents Fel d 1–induced mediator release and signaling events in basophils obtained from cat allergic patients.

Food allergy is a major health problem. In the next article of the third set, Nowak-Wegrzyn discusses novel aspects of native and recombinant food proteins in the treatment of food allergies. The article begins with a state-of-the-art approach to a patient who has a food allergy, followed by a detailed table that highlights the current worldwide experience in oral food desensitization. Significant successes of immunotherapy in the food allergy world are described, such as the ability of subcutaneous peanut immunotherapy and birch immunotherapy to reduce the severity of peanut allergy and apple allergy, respectively. She describes the successful use of oral and sublingual immunotherapy and of native, recombinant, and engineered recombinant allergens administered in bacterial adjuvant to prevent allergy in mice.

The final article of the third set is a provocative rice-based vaccine strategy of inducing oral tolerance to prevent specific allergies. Here Fumio Takaiwa describes how T cell epitopes in Cry j 1 and Cry j 2 Japanese cedar allergy were identified. These epitopes were cloned into a soybean protein gene as a fusion protein gene and transferred into the rice genome. Feeding mice this transgenic rice grain expressing Cry j T cell eiptopes prevented Th2 and IgE allergic responses to Japanese cedar challenge. Takaiwa describes how their group developed a "human version" of transgenic rice that had multiple human dominant T cell epitopes, and demonstrated that feeding mice that specifically recognize only a specific Cry j 1 epitope prevents allergies.

These articles summarize some aspects of an ever-increasing array of fascinating studies in this emerging field. As we learn more about allergic proteins, lipids, and carbohydrates through experimental and computational methods, it is highly likely that the information will be "translated" into additional novel and provocative vaccines that will reduce allergies and asthma in the foreseeable future. Perhaps some day in the not-too-distant future, it may be possible to feed a cocktail of different "allergen-specific cereal" to children born in atopic families, thereby preventing development of allergies altogether.

I hope this issue of the *Immunology and Allergy Clinics of North America* is useful to students, postgraduates, allergists, and scientists throughout the world. I would like to acknowledge the Consulting Editor, Rafeul Alam, for inviting me to serve as Guest Editor for this issue and for his valuable input, to my scientific colleagues who spent their time and effort to write articles for this issue, and to Carla Holloway for her outstanding editorial support.

Finally, I wish to acknowledge my parents, Bimal and Gouri Sur, for giving me the values required to focus my life on a career in science.

Sanjiv Sur, MD
Division of Allergy, Immunology, and Pulmonary
University of Texas Medical Branch
301 University Boulevard, MRB 8.104
Galveston, TX 77555, USA

E-mail address: sasur@utmb.edu

ELSEVIER
SAUNDERS

Immunol Allergy Clin N Am
27 (2007) 1–27

IMMUNOLOGY
AND ALLERGY
CLINICS
OF NORTH AMERICA

Bioinformatics Approaches to Classifying Allergens and Predicting Cross-Reactivity

Catherine H. Schein, PhD[a,b], Ovidiu Ivanciuc, PhD[a], Werner Braun, PhD[a,*]

[a]*Sealy Center for Structural Biology and Molecular Biophysics, Department of Biochemistry and Molecular Biology, University of Texas Medical Branch, 301 University Boulevard, Galveston, TX 77555-0857, USA*
[b]*Department of Microbiology and Immunology, University of Texas Medical Branch, 301 University Boulevard, Galveston, TX 77555-0857, USA*

Allergy is a steadily increasing health problem for all age groups in the United States. Food allergies, mostly against milk, eggs, peanuts, soy, or wheat, affect up to 8% of infants and young children [1–3]. In addition, many allergies to food (including shellfish, nuts, and fruits) and air-borne particulate matter (such as insect residue and tree and grass pollens) can develop later in life. One hypothesis is that this late onset may be the result of individuals being sensitized by long-term exposure to environmental factors that contain proteins similar to those in the known triggers of allergenic response [1,4–6]. Recent studies have identified common molecular features of proteins from different sources, which could account for clinically important cross-reactivity [7,8] and sensitivity [9,10]. For example, major allergenic proteins in peanut have been isolated and peptides from their sequences that react with IgE from patient sera identified [6,11,12]. Proteins similar to these allergens were subsequently found in other foods that are known to elicit clinically significant responses in individuals with peanut allergies [13], such as tree nuts [14], soy [15], and legumes [16,17].

This work was supported by grants from the Food and Drug Administration (FD-U-002249), the Texas Higher Education Coordinating Board (ATP grant 004952-0036-2003), the National Institute of Health (R01 AI 064913) and the U.S. Environmental Protection Agency under a STAR Research Assistance Agreement (No. RD 833137). The article has not been formally reviewed by the EPA, and the views expressed in this document are solely those of the authors.

* Corresponding author.
E-mail address: webraun@utmb.edu (W. Braun).

doi:10.1016/j.iac.2006.11.005 ***immunology.theclinics.com***

To show how valuable comparing the proteins that are known to cause allergy can be, allergens classified as pathogenesis-related proteins have extremely conserved sequences in many different plants [18–21]. Some sources of allergens belonging to pathogenesis-related proteins of group 5 (PR5) are shown in Fig. 1. The first allergen in this group was isolated from cedar pollen [22,23], but related proteins bound to IgE from patients allergic to cherries, bell pepper, apple, and tomato were subsequently identified [24]. Because the sources of these closely related allergenic proteins are so different, sensitive individuals may feel that they are experiencing multiple allergy syndrome, when they actually may have a strong reaction to one protein type that is found in many sources. Therefore, by identifying the common protein using the bioinformatics tools described in this article, more specific treatments can be defined [25].

Allergenic proteins from pollens, particularly from cedar [22,26–28], birch [29–31], and grass [32–35] are similar in overall sequence and structure. Other families of allergenic proteins have been isolated from primary food

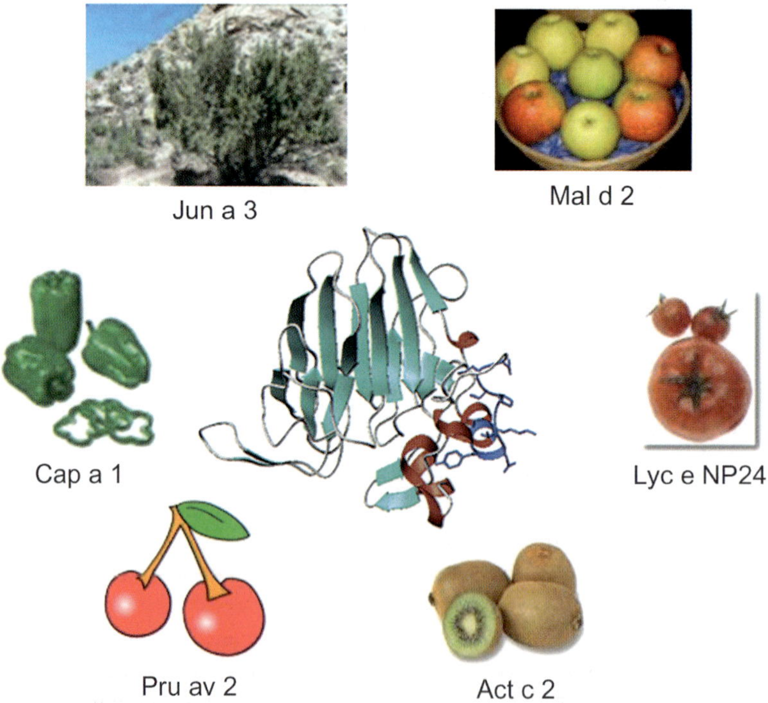

Fig. 1. Different products can contain similar allergenic proteins. In this case, an allergen, Jun a 3, originally isolated from the pollen of mountain cedar was found to be a member of the PR5 family of proteins, and was modeled based on its similarity to a protein of known structure, thaumatin. Subsequently, similar allergenic proteins were isolated from many food plants, including bell pepper (Cap a 1), cherry (Pru av 2), kiwi (Act c 2), tomato (Lyc e NP24), and apple (Mal d 2).

sources, such as milk [36–38] (casein [37,39,40] and lactoglobulin [41–43]), egg [44] (ovomucoid [45–47] and lysozyme [48]), shrimp and related species (tropomyosins [49–51]), fish (parvalbumin [52–54]), and legumes (albumins [55–58] and glycinins [59–61]).

Many allergens in pollen and fruits have similar sequences and structures, as shown in Fig. 1. Identifying the protein group can be used to guide specific immunotherapy. For example, clinically important cross-reactivities between birch pollen and several different types of fruits could be accounted for by showing that they contain similar proteins [62–66]. In a group of patients who had oral allergy syndrome to apples and birch pollen sensitivity, the root cause was hypothesized to be the similarity between the allergen Bet v 1 and the apple protein Mal d 1. Specific immunotherapy with a Bet v 1–containing extract was able to mitigate sensitivity to this fruit [67].

These successes explain the current interest in developing bioinformatics approaches to interpret the accumulated body of knowledge about the proteins that elicit severe IgE-mediated reactions [8,68–70]. Until recently, much of the information about allergens was distributed in many different literature sources, making oversight and direct sequence comparisons difficult, especially for clinicians managing patients directly [71]. However, several databases are now available that contain sequences and information about allergenic proteins (Table 1). This article discusses the specific features in each of these databases and highlights how the Structural Database of Allergenic Proteins (SDAP) (http://fermi.utmb.edu/SDAP/) [72,73] can be used to compare the sequence, structure, and epitopes of allergens. SDAP has been designed to be user-friendly and to be of maximum use to clinicians and scientists interested in determining the molecular basis of allergen cross-reactivity [13,24,74].

Database approaches to classifying allergenic proteins

Overview of allergen databases

Table 1 lists public databases dedicated to allergens, the URL addresses, and their features. Most of these databases are simply lists of allergenic proteins or sources, with limited cross-indexing. For example, the International Union of Immunological Societies (IUIS) site, available at: http://www.allergen.org, simply lists alphabetically the official names of all the proteins this organization recognizes as allergens. The tables contain brief information for each allergen, such as source, references, and Genbank accession numbers for the sequence. However, no cross-indexing is available, and therefore relationships between proteins are difficult to identify. Another database, AllAllergy (http://allallergy.net/), is a collection of links for allergy-related Internet sites, which can be useful for obtaining clinical information, organizations, publications, events, and databases. Other recent reviews provide more details on general allergy databases [25,71].

Table 1
Web sites with information about allergens, allergen databases, and allergenicity prediction servers

Web site	URL	Information available
Nomenclature and general information databases		
AllAllergy	http://allallergy.net/	A portal to allergy information, useful for the general public
IUIS (International Union of Immunological Societies)	http://www.allergen.org	List of official names, grouped by source, and Genbank accession numbers of allergens
Allergome	http://www.allergome.org	List of official names of allergens, and links to PubMed & sequence databases
CSL (Central Science Laboratory, UK)	http://www.csl.gov.uk/allergen/index.htm	List of official names of allergens with sequence links to Genbank
National Center for Food Safety and Technology	http://www.iit.edu/~sgendel/fa.htm	List of official names of food allergens with links to Genbank
Protall	http://www.ifrn.bbsrc.ac.uk/protall/	Allergen names, plus links to detailed biochemical, structural, and clinical data
InformAll	http://foodallergens.ifr.ac.uk/	Biochemical information, mainly for food allergens, epitopes, sequences, links to literature
Cross-referenced databases with tools to compare sequences		
FARRP	http://allergenonline.com/asp/public/login.asp	List of official names of allergens, sequence links to Genbank, and a FASTA search for related sequences
ADFS – Allergen Database for Food Safety	http://allergen.nihs.go.jp/ADFS/	Allergen sequences, implements the WHO allergenicity rules using FASTA
Cross-referenced databases with tools for prediction of allergenicity		
SDAP (Structural database of Allergenic proteins) and SDAP-FOOD	http://fermi.utmb.edu/SDAP	Allergen sequences, on-site and cross-referenced by source and protein type, with links to all major sequence and structural databases, IgE epitopes collection, tools for sequence and epitope comparison, on-site information about experimental structures of allergens, and high-quality protein models

Table 1 (*continued*)

Web site	URL	Information available
ALLERDB	http://sdmc.i2r.a-star.edu.sg/Templar/DB/Allergen/	List of official names of allergens, a BLAST search, and implements the WHO allergenicity rules
Web servers for allergenicity prediction		
WebAllergen	http://weballergen.bii.a-star.edu.sg/	Predicts the potential allergenicity of proteins using motifs found by a wavelet algorithm
Allermatch	www.allermatch.org/	Implements the WHO allergenicity rules using FASTA
AlgPred	http://www.imtech.res.in/raghava/algpred/	Predicts allergenicity with MEME/MAST motifs

Abbreviations: ALLERDB, Allergen Database; BLAST, basic local alignment search tool; MEME, Multiple Em for Motif Elicitation.

Other databases are cross-indexed and much more useful for experts wanting to identify cross-reacting allergens and their natural sources. Allergome (http://www.allergome.org) is a comprehensive database of clinical, biologic, and structural information about IUIS and non-IUIS–recognized allergens. Allergome records the name, source, biochemical, and immunochemical features for each allergen, but no computational tools are integrated in this database. Stadler and Stadler [75] introduced the Multiple Em for Motif Elicitation (MEME) motifs for allergens, which are included in Allergome. Unlike IgE epitopes that are discussed later, these motifs are long and could be more properly called conserved domains in the sequences of closely related allergens.

Another database, maintained by the Central Science Laboratory, UK (CSL) (http://www.csl.gov.uk/allergen/index.htm), lists official names of allergens with sequence links to Genbank. This database is similar to the Biotechnology Information for Food Safety Database (National Center for Food Safety and Technology, http://www.iit.edu/~sgendel/fa.htm), which provides comprehensive lists of allergens with links to sequences from the Protein Information Resource (PIR), SwissProt, and Genbank. The Protall project (http://www.ifrn.bbsrc.ac.uk/protall/) developed a database of plant food allergens that contains links to detailed biochemical, structural, and clinical data. The development of the Protall database has been part of the InformAll project since 2001 (http://foodallergens.ifr.ac.uk/).

A few databases allow direct comparison of allergen sequences using conventional search tools, and permit the use of the World Health Organization (WHO) guidelines for predicting potential allergenicity [76]. These guidelines specify that a protein might cross-react with an allergen if it is at least 35% identical over a frame of 80 amino acids, or contains an exact match of any peptide of 6 to 8 amino acids with the allergen [77]. The Food Allergy Research and Resource Program (FARRP) database (http://allergenonline.com/asp/public/login.asp) contains a searchable list of allergens, sequence links to Genbank, and a FASTA search for related sequences. The Allergen Database for Food Safety (ADFS) (http://allergen.nihs.go.jp/ADFS/) contains allergen sequences and epitope information, and implements the WHO allergenicity rules using FASTA. Allergen Database (ALLERDB) (http://sdmc.i2r.a-star.edu.sg/Templar/DB/Allergen/) lists official names of allergens, has a basic logic alignment search tool (BLAST), and provides a sequence comparison tool that implements the WHO guidelines.

Overview of the Structural Database of Allergenic Proteins

Methods to check for how well a test protein matches any allergen, according to the WHO guidelines, are also implemented in the SDAP [72,73]. Unlike the publicly available allergen databases discussed previously, SDAP has integrated search tools to allow users to rapidly compare the molecular properties of allergenic proteins and their epitopes. In addition, SDAP contains special tools that were developed to compare short sequences, and these tools permit rapid identification of allergens that contain sequences statistically similar to known linear IgE epitopes [13,24]. SDAP was developed for basic research on the nature of allergenic proteins, and to allow regulatory agencies, food scientists, and physicians to determine if a novel protein has allergenic potential. No special training is needed to access the data, and the tools are implemented in a user-friendly fashion. Searches are direct and rapid, and therefore can be performed from a computer in a clinic with Internet access.

SDAP contains information on sequence, three-dimensional structures, and epitopes of known allergens from published literature and compiled databases on the Web [72,73]. The major uses of SDAP for clinicians are to determine food sources that could induce cross-reactions in sensitive individuals and to help prepare dietary recommendations for patients who have allergies and a known sensitivity. For example, patients who have a food allergy can be advised to avoid other foods that contain proteins similar to the ones that are known to trigger an allergic reaction. Alternatively, a recombinant protein can be used to determine the scope of the allergic response and to suggest candidates for specific immunotherapy.

The basic structure of the Structural Database of Allergenic Proteins

The best way to learn using SDAP is to go to the Web site and open the main search page, which has a link to a list of all the allergenic proteins in the database. Selecting an allergen of interest (eg, Asp f 1, which is a major fungal allergen) opens a new descriptive page for that allergen. This page contains a summary of all the data archived in SDAP for that allergen, including the official name (according to the IUIS Web site listing, http://www.allergen.org/); the scientific and common names for the species; general source of the allergens; allergen type; species; systematic name; brief description; sequence accession numbers from SwissProt, PIR, and the National Center for Biotechnology Information (NCBI); and, where available, the program database file name for a structure. All of this information is cross-referenced to the original data sources, which can be directly accessed by clicking on the links from each allergen page.

Allergenic proteins belong to discrete groups, or families, of structures. SDAP has several different methods for comparing the sequences of allergens within the database. The in-house bioinformatics methods permit almost instantaneous sequence similarity searching, with direct connections to much larger databases. To determine what other sequences are similar to the amino acid sequence of an allergen, one can perform full-length sequences for similarity to the known allergens by selecting the BLAST and FASTA [78] searches. These searches can be activated directly from the main descriptive page for any of the allergens in SDAP of known sequence.

The Pfam grouping, discussed in more detail later, is available for most of the allergens in SDAP and rapidly indicates which other allergens a given protein resembles. Links to structural models for the various allergens allow three-dimensional visualization of common areas of the proteins. Another box on the allergen page indicates what IgE epitopes are known, and each sequence is linked to tools that can be used to automatically identify similar or identical sequences in all other sequences in SDAP. Other tools allow users to map the IgE-containing peptides onto the experimental modeled structures of allergens. Fig. 2 shows two examples of this tool, where the IgE epitopes of two fungal allergens Asp f 1 and Asp f 3 have been mapped on an experimentally determined structure (Protein Data Bank [PDB] 1AQZ) and on the Modeling Package (MPACK) (http://curie.utmb.edu/mpack/) model, respectively.

SDAP is also integrated with other bioinformatics servers, allowing users to investigate structural similarity and neighbors using the Structural Classification of Proteins (SCOP) database [79]; the Topology of Protein Structure (TOPS) database [80]; the Class, Architecture, Topology, and Homologous superfamily (CATH) classification [81]; Combinatorial Extension (CE) of the optimal path [82]; the Families of Structurally Similar Proteins (FSSP) database [83]; and the Vector Alignment Search Tool (VAST) [84].

Epitope lists for allergenic proteins

SDAP is a unique allergen data source because it contains lists of IgE-binding epitopes of allergenic proteins assembled from the primary literature. Most of these sequence segments have been identified through in vitro binding to short peptides on solid phases that are assumed to represent epitopes

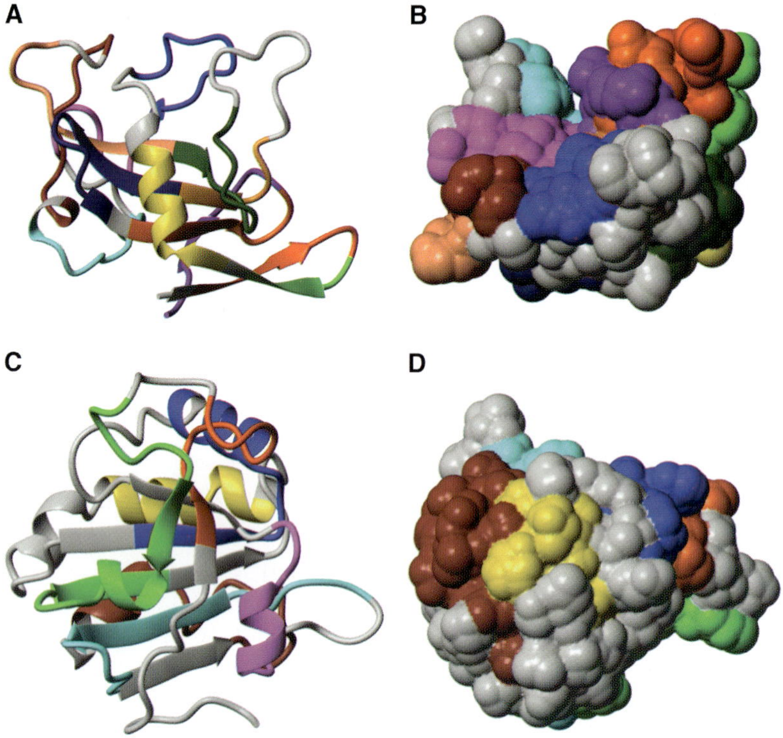

Fig. 2. IgE epitopes mapped on the experimental structure (PDB 1AQZ) of Asp f 1 (*A* and *B*) and our MPACK model of Asp f 3 (*C* and *D*), two allergens from the fungus causing aspergillosis.

that may be involved in eliciting allergic reactions. In a few cases, the biologic importance of the identified epitopes has been tested; for example through mutating these areas and showing that the IgE-binding capacity was thereby diminished [85–87] or that the isolated peptides can interfere with antibody binding to the whole protein [27,28]. Currently, IgE epitope information is available for 27 allergens in SDAP: fungi (Alt a 1, Asp f 1, Asp f 2, Asp f 3, Asp f 13, Pen ch 18), pollen from Texas mountain cedar (Jun a 1, Jun a 3) and related species (Cha o 1, Cry j 1, Cry j 2), weed pollen (Par j 1, Par j 2), rubber (Hev b 1, Hev b 3, Hev b 5), yellowjacket venom (Ves v 5), peanut (Ara h 1, Ara h 2, Ara h 3), buckwheat (Fag e 1), hen egg (Gal d 1), soybean (Gly m glycinin G1, Gly m glycinin G2), English walnut (Jug r 1), and shrimp (Pen a 1, Pen i 1).

The authors developed special methodology for finding homologues of known epitopes in the sequences of other SDAP entries: the property distance (*PD*) search, which is later discussed in detail. The *PD* distance method was developed specifically to detect meaningful similarities when comparing short sequences [72,73]. *PD* searches can show similarities in IgE epitope sequences, even from different allergenic proteins [13,24].

FASTA for comparing the overall sequences of allergenic proteins

The first step in determining whether proteins are potentially cross-reactive is to determine their overall sequence similarity to other allergens using FASTA [78]. FASTA can be run automatically from any sequence file in SDAP with a mouse-click, and outputs a table that lists all similar allergens in SDAP with their expectation value (E-value). Table 2 is an example of a FASTA search result in SDAP for the cedar pollen allergen Jun a 3. The last column of Table 2 lists the E-value that indicates the statistical significance of the hit. The E-value is a measure of how many matches with the same sequence similarity would be expected to occur randomly in a database of a given size. Therefore, a low E-value (eg, less than 10^{-6}) indicates a high significance of the sequence match.

Note that the most similar entry in SDAP for Jun a 3 (ie, the one with the lowest E-value) is another pathogenesis-related protein (group 5) from a related cypress tree, Cup a 3. However, similar allergenic proteins have been isolated from various vegetables and fruits, which are shown pictorially in Fig. 1. Based on these FASTA alignments, one can anticipate that someone with severe cedar pollen allergy might also develop oral allergy symptoms [88,89] when eating apples or cherries, for example. In addition to those mentioned earlier, other clinically relevant cross-reactivities have been shown, such as those linking dust mite sensitization and the development of food allergies to shrimp and other crustaceans. This cross-reactivity is believed to be based on the similarities of the tropomyosins in these organisms [72,73,88].

Nomenclature and classes of allergenic proteins

The Structural Database of Allergenic Proteins can help determine names for newly identified allergens

Names of allergens are only official after they are approved by the IUIS. Submitted allergenic proteins are named using a thorough process, agreed to

Table 2
Output of an automatic FASTA search in Structural Database of Allergenic Proteins

No	Allergen	Sequence	Source	Sequence length	Bit score	E-score
1	Jun a 3	P81295	cedar pollen	225	311.0	1.0e-86
2	Cup a 3	CAC05258	cypress	199	272.9	2.7e-75
3	Cap a 1w	CAC34055	bell pepper	246	167.5	1.7e-43
4	Lyc e NP24	P12670	tomato	247	161.2	1.4e-41
5	Cap a 1	AAG34078	bell pepper	180	136.2	3.4e-34
6	Mal d 2	CAC10270	apple	246	77.0	3.0e-16
7	Pru av 2	P50694	cherry	245	75.1	1.2e-15
8	Act c 2	P81370	kiwi	29	36.0	7.9e-05

This search started from the file for the allergen Jun a 3, an allergen isolated from cedar pollen. This PR5 protein is related (ie, the sequence match has an E-score <0.01) to seven other allergenic proteins in SDAP.

by the member societies. Allergens are named by abbreviating the Latin name of the species from which they were isolated (eg, *Cryptomeria japonica* becomes Cry j) followed by a number that indicates the order in which they were identified (Cry j 1, a vicilin related to Jun a 1 from *Juniperus ashei* and similar allergens from other Taxaceae). After the original rounds of naming, the committee has tried, when possible, to maintain a structural or functional relationship across related taxa in the allergen numbering system. In the ideal case, the number would also be consistent with the protein class of the allergen. Thus, the PR5-related allergens in cypress pollens, regardless of species, would be number 3 (Cry j 3, Jun a 3). However, the numbering is not always consistent, and the PR5 allergens from apple, cherry, and bell pepper are Mal d 2, Pru av 2, and Cap a 1, respectively. Used at an early stage in the nomenclature process, SDAP can provide enough information to determine rapidly what other related allergens have similar sequences, and thus should have the same number.

Routine use of SDAP can prevent certain problems, such as those that may arise when discoverers of a new allergen give it a name based on their understanding of how many other allergens have been previously isolated from the given biologic source. Although the IUIS may change this name, once a protein has been named in the literature, obtaining wide acceptance of a different designation is often difficult [90]. For example, an allergen identified in *Juniper oxycedrus* was originally called Jun o 2 by its discoverer. However, when the IUIS examined this allergen, they realized that this was a different protein from the other cypress allergens named type 2, such as Jun a 2 and Cyp a 2 (Table 3). Therefore, they assigned the protein the official name of Jun o 4 [91], with relevance to its similarity to the Bet v 4 protein of birch pollen (see lower part of Table 3). SDAP names this protein Jun o 4, but alerts users who type in Jun o 2 of the name change because other databases, including PIR, GenBank, and Swissprot, continue to identify Jun o 4 as Jun o 2. If the SDAP had been used initially to name this allergen, this confusing situation (which will get worse if a real Jun o 2 is isolated) would not have occurred.

The other feature of allergen nomenclature illustrated by Table 3 is that allergens with closely related sequences, such as those in the bottom section of the table, can have widely differing numbers. Furthermore, the names of closely related proteins can differ. For example, food allergens are generally categorized as seed storage proteins or albumins. Depending on their degree of identity to other proteins, they may be additionally categorized as vicilins, proglycinins, 7S albumin, or another designation, which can then determine the common name of the allergen. Because a radically different nomenclature scheme is unlikely to be introduced in the near future, database searches such as this one will provide the best way to truly indicate which allergens are most related.

Grouping allergenic proteins according to major Pfam families

Classifying allergens into functional groups of proteins can indicate important relationships, and structural and sequence groupings allow experts to

Table 3
Results of two automatic FASTA searches in Structural Database of Allergen Proteins that illustrate how to use this site to correctly name a new allergen

No	Allergen	Sequence link in SwissProt/NCBI/PIR	Sequence length	Bit score	E-score
Search with Jun a 2					
1	Jun a 2	CAC05582	507	794.0	0.0e+00
2	Cry j 2	P43212	514	579.2	9.5e-167
4	Phl p 13	CAB42886	394	198.8	2.4e-52
Search with Jun o 4					
1	Jun o 4	064943	165	229.0	2.7e-62
2	Ole e 8	Q9M7R0	171	89.8	2.2e-20
4	Syr v 3	P58171	81	62.5	1.7e-12
5	Bra n 2	BAA09633	82	61.3	4.0e-12
7	Bra r 2	Q39406	83	61.3	4.0e-12
8	Aln g 4	081701	85	61.3	4.1e-12
9	Bet v 4	Q39419	85	60.9	5.4e-12
11	Ole e 3	081092	84	59.6	1.3e-11
12	Phl p 7	082040	78	58.8	2.2e-11
15	Bra n 1	Q42470	79	52.8	1.4e-09
16	Bra r 1	Q42470	79	52.8	1.4e-09
17	Bet v 3	P43187	205	35.8	4.9e-04
18	Gad c 1	P02622	113	34.9	4.9e-04
19	Sal s 1	Q91482	109	33.6	1.1e-03
20	Sco j 1	P59747	109	31.3	5.5e-03

Although the cedar pollen allergens Jun a 2 and Cry j 2 are very close in sequence (ie, have a very low E-value), they are not related to the allergen originally called Jun o 2. This protein, officially named Jun o 4 by the IUIS, is similar to Bet v 4 and other allergens of that sequence family.

identify significant similarities in proteins with different names. These structural similarities may also underlie functional similarities that are probably not related to the allergenic potential of the protein [74]. The most common protein groups for plant allergens are cupin, prolamin, and plant defense proteins. Representative allergens from the cupin superfamily are vicilin and legumin from tree nuts, peanuts, and soybean. Important allergens from the prolamin superfamily are amylase and protease inhibitors, nonspecific lipid transfer proteins (LTPs), and 2S albumin seed storage proteins. Plant defense proteins comprise allergens from several classes, such as pathogenesis-related proteins, proteases, and protease inhibitors [8,89,92].

Users of SDAP can identify allergens that are significantly similar to one another according to their Pfam or enzyme classification. Pfam (http://www.sanger.ac.uk/Software/Pfam/) is a list of multiple sequence alignments of related protein domains, classified in two ways. The Pfam-A database lists protein families that are grouped by their common function and sequence, using expert knowledge and experimental data. Pfam-B is computer-generated and contains alignments of proteins sequences selected based on a minimum level of sequence identity, regardless of their protein function. Most

SDAP entries have now been classified to one of these groupings. Easy access to this Pfam classification for any allergen can be accessed from the "List SDAP" menu item.

The most common Pfam families for allergens are listed in Table 4, where 18 Pfam families are shown that have between 34 and 7 allergens each. The most common Pfam families for allergens are PF00234 (protease inhibitor/seed storage/LTP family, 34 allergens), PF00235 (profilins, 27 allergens), PF00036 (EF hand, 23 allergens), and PF01357 (pollen allergen, 20 allergens). Table 5 lists allergens from these four Pfam families, with representative structures shown in Fig. 3 (Pru p 3 from PF00234, Hev b 8 from PF00235, Bet v 4 from PF00036, and Phl p 2 from PF01357).

Computational methods for predicting cross-reactivity

Cross-reactive allergenic proteins are usually very similar in sequence and structure at the molecular level, regardless of their source. Most allergens can be grouped into discrete sequence families according to their Pfam classification. However, a typical Pfam will contain allergenic and nonallergenic proteins. Quantitatively discriminating the allergenic members in a group of similar proteins is a difficult task, and one that eludes the programs currently implemented in popular databases. Experimentally, cross-reactive allergens typically have high sequence identity, which can drop to as low as 35% (hence the WHO guidelines). Still, point mutations are known to eliminate IgE binding [5,14,30,85], as shown by the example of isoforms of Bet v 1, which are 98% identical but are not cross-reactive [93–95]. For this reason, the results

Table 4
The most abundant Pfam A allergen families from Structural Database of Allergen Proteins

Pfam code	Family name	No. of allergens
PF00234	Protease inhibitor/seed storage/LTP family	34
PF00235	Profilin	27
PF00036	EF hand	23
PF01357	Pollen allergen	20
PF00188	SCP-like extracellular protein	19
PF00407	Pathogenesis-related protein Bet v I family	16
PF00190	Cupin	15
PF00261	Tropomyosin	15
PF00061	Lipocalin/cytosolic fatty-acid binding protein family	12
PF03330	Rare lipoprotein A (RlpA)-like double-psi beta-barrel	12
PF00042	Globin	9
PF00544	Pectate lyase	9
PF00112	Papain family cysteine protease	8
PF00428	60s Acidic ribosomal protein	8
PF00082	Subtilase family	7
PF00314	Thaumatin family	7
PF01190	Pollen proteins Ole e I family	7
PF01620	Ribonuclease (pollen allergen)	7

Table 5
Allergens from the four most populated with allergens Pfam families

PF00234: Protease inhibitor/seed storage/LTP family					
Amb a 6	Ana o 3	Ara h 2	Ara h 6	Ber e 1	Bra j 1
Bra n 1	Cor a 8	Fag e 8kD	Gly m 1	Hev b 12	Hor v 1
Hor v 21	Jug n 1	Jug r 1	Lyc e 3	Mal d 3	Ory s TAI
Par j 1	Par j 2	Pru ar 3	Pru av 3	Pru d 3	Pru p 3
Pyr c 3	Ric c 1	Ses i 1	Ses i 2	Sin a 1	Tri a gliadin
Tri a glutenin	Tri a TAI	Vit v 1	Zea m 14	—	—
PF00235: Profilin					
Ana c 1	Api g 4	Ara h 5	Ara t 8	Bet v 2	Cap a 2
Che a 2	Cor a 2	Cuc m 2	Cyn d 12	Dau c 4	Gly m 3
Hel a 2	Hev b 8	Lit c 1	Lyc e 1	Mal d 4	Mer a 1
Mus xp 1	Ole e 2	Par j 3	Phl p 11	Phl p 12	Pru av 4
Pru p 4	Pyr c 4	Tri a profilin	—	—	—
PF00036: EF hand					
Aln g 4	Bet v 3	Bet v 4	Bos d 3	Bra n 1	Bra n 2
Bra r 1	Che a 3	Cyn d 7	Cyp c 1	Gad c 1	Gad m 1
Hom s 4	Jun o 4	Ole e 3	Ole e 8	Phl p 7	Ran e 1
Ran e 2	Sal s 1	Sco j 1	Syr v 3	The c 1	—
PF01357: Pollen allergen					
Ara t expansin	Cyn d 1	Cyn d 15	Cyn d 2	Dac g 2	Dac g 3
Gly m 2	Hol l 1	Lol p 1	Lol p 2	Lol p 3	Ory s 1
Pan s 1	Pha a 1	Phl p 1	Phl p 2	Poa p a	Tri a 3
Tri a ps93	Zea m 1	—	—	—	—

of current methods for predicting the allergenicity of a given protein should be considered cautiously. The general consensus of a recent International Bioinformatics Workshop Meeting [96] on this problem concluded that more detailed statistical analysis of the properties of allergenic proteins versus nonallergens is needed and that numerical benchmarks for prediction methods should be developed. The current methodology is described and other methods are outlined later, based on identifying motifs of allergenic protein groups, that may have more success in defining cross-reactive allergens and areas for potential IgE recognition. Some of the more advanced methods implemented in SDAP for comparing IgE epitopes are emphasized, because this is one of the key features of the database that can be used in the future to design allergen vaccines and proteins with reduced allergenic potential.

Testing automatic computational procedures for allergenicity prediction

One of the most difficult tasks in allergen recognition is to distinguish features of proteins that are allergenic from closely related proteins that are not [97]. The tropomyosin family is a particularly difficult problem, because the allergenic members of the family, such as Der p10 from dust mite and Met e 1 from shrimp, are highly identical to mammalian tropomyosins that are not

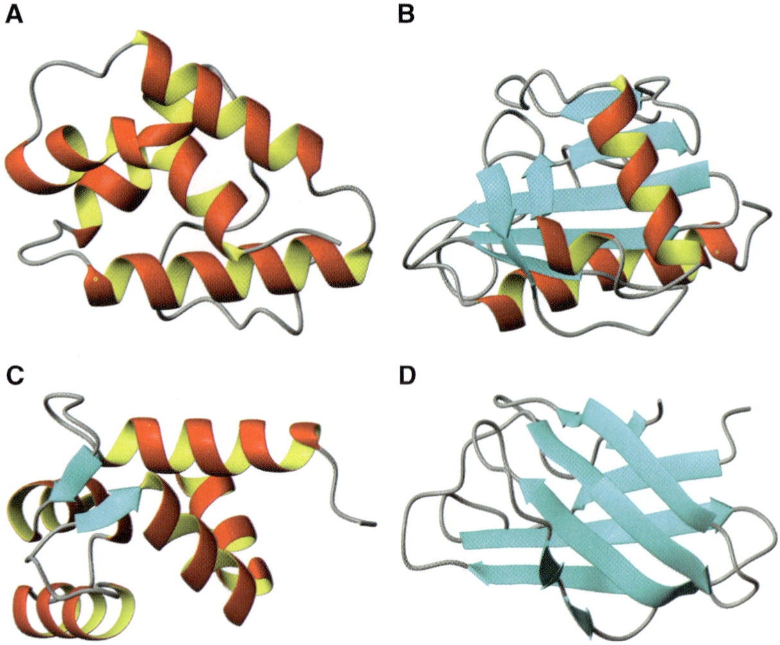

Fig. 3. PDB structures for allergens from the four most abundant Pfam families: (*A*) Pru p 3 (PF00234, protease inhibitor/seed storage/LTP family); (*B*) Hev b 8 (PF00235, profilin); (*C*) Bet v 4 (PF00036, EF hand); and (*D*) Phl p 2 (PF01357, pollen allergen).

allergenic. The authors tested the ability of three allergenicity prediction servers (WebAllergen, Allermatch, and AlgPred) to discriminate between four nonallergenic tropomyosins from animal sources and four allergenic tropomyosins from insects and shellfish (Table 6). The first server, WebAllergen [98], found that all the tropomyosins have five wavelet allergenic motifs [99] in common, whereas the allergenic tropomyosins have a few additional wavelet motifs that distinguish them. These findings are promising, if these allergenic motifs could also be shown to contain IgE-binding areas.

However, other rapid methods were unable to discriminate the two groups at all. Allermatch, which applies the FAO/WHO allergenicity guidelines, predicts that all eight tropomyosins are allergens. The authors also tested the MEME classifier based on motifs identified in groups of allergenic proteins [75]. This method, as implemented in the AlgPred server, predicted that all eight tropomyosins are nonallergens. Besides the MEME classification approach, the AlgPred server evaluates the allergenicity through scanning for known IgE epitopes, performing a BLAST search, using a support vector machines (SVM) prediction based on amino acid or dipeptide composition, and with a hybrid approach that combines the above five procedures [100]. The SVM dipeptide composition classifier predicts that all eight tropomyosins are allergens.

Table 6
Test of three allergenicity prediction servers

			Allermatch	AlgPred	AlgPred
Tropomyosin	SwissProt	WebAllergen	FAO/WHO	MEME	SVM dipeptide
Human	TPM1_HUMAN	6 motifs: 13, 15, 25, 26, 30, 31	Y	N	Y
Bovine	Q5KR49_BOVIN	6 motifs: 13, 15, 25, 26, 30, 31	Y	N	Y
Pig	TPM1_PIG	6 motifs: 13, 14, 15, 26, 30, 31	Y	N	Y
Chicken	TPM1_CHICK	7 motifs: 13, 14, 15, 25, 26, 30, 31	Y	N	Y
Der p 10, house dust mite	TPM_DERPT	10 motifs: 13, 14, 15, 16, 25, 26, 29, 30, 31, 55	Y	N	Y
Per a 7 American cockroach	TPM_PERAM	10 motifs: 13, 14, 15, 25, 26, 29, 30, 31, 55, 7	Y	N	Y
Met e 1 sand shrimp	TPM_METEN	9 motifs: 13, 14, 15, 25, 26, 30, 31, 55, 7	Y	N	Y
Ani s 3 herring worm	TPM_ANISI	9 motifs: 13, 14, 15, 25, 26, 29, 30, 31, 55	Y	N	Y

Three database prediction methods are unable to discriminate the allergenic sequences from insects shellfish (*bottom four sequences*) from the nonallergenic tropomyosins from animals (*top sequences*). The former proteins do, however, contain motifs that are not present in the latter.

Consistent with earlier results [101,102], the WHO guidelines implemented in allergenicity prediction servers seem unable to discriminate between closely related proteins, such as the nonallergenic and allergenic tropomyosins, because their overall sequences are too similar. However, other studies have shown that these guidelines are useful for detecting proteins that are sufficiently similar to known allergens with which they might cross-react [103]. Several reports show that the succession of bioinformatics and experimental procedures from the FAO/WHO decision tree may be valuable in investigating the protein allergenicity [104–106].

Efforts to improve correlations based on the whole protein sequence are ongoing. Methods based on analyzing the statistics of FASTA alignments with machine learning procedures have been tested [107,108]. In one case, such an algorithm was able to correctly classify 81% of 91 food allergens and 98% of 367 nonallergens [109]. This level of accuracy could make the method useful for clinically discriminating protein groups to be avoided by patients who have a known sensitivity to a related protein.

Another alternative is to detect discrete areas of a protein sequence similar to known IgE epitopes. The SDAP list of IgE epitopes, most of which were identified through IgE recognition of linear arrays of synthetic peptides, is unique, as are the tools incorporated at the site for detecting identical and similar sequences (the *PD* tool) in other known allergens.

Motif-based methods for allergenicity prediction

Alternatively, one can define discrete areas of residue conservation, or *motifs*, in related allergenic proteins of known clinical cross-reactivity as possible areas for IgE binding. Several groups have defined conserved sequences in groups of allergens [75,99,102,110]. This article defines a motif as an area of sequence that is extremely conserved in a group of related proteins. Although motifs can be long, for the practical purpose of defining areas likely to be IgE epitopes, a normal length is between 6 and 15 amino acids. The authors look for areas where the side chains show conserved physical–chemical properties (PCPs), such as hydrophobicity, size, or alpha-helical propensity, rather than strict identify. The underlying assumption is that for a group of cross-reactive allergenic proteins, the IgE epitope areas will have common PCPs. The authors' method begins by aligning the sequences of known allergens that are related to one another, such as those in the tropomyosin or vicilin family. The PCPMer suite (available at http://landau.utmb.edu:8080/WebPCPMer/HomePage/index.html) finds sequence motifs in protein families by identifying regions with highly conserved PCPs. These PCP motifs are determined by conserving the five quantitative property vectors E_1 through E_5, which summarize many different physicochemical properties of the side chains of the amino acids, including size, hydrophobicity, and tendency to form helical or strand secondary structures [111,112]. The descriptors E_1 to E_5 were determined by multidimensional scaling of 237 of these PCPs, and encode numerically the maximum distance between the various side chains in a five-dimensional space. These descriptors are also the basis of the PD scale for classifying sequences similar to known IgE epitopes, as described later.

Other efforts to predict allergenicity were directed toward identifying linear epitopes [113]. Saha and Raghava [114] used a recurrent neural network for the prediction of continuous B-cell epitopes. Although short amino acid sequence matches seem to have little value for allergenicity prediction [115], peptide motifs common to groups of allergens may be a better way to distinguish allergens. An efficient machine learning classification scheme, based on identifying a set of allergen-representative peptides that appear in allergens but have a low or no occurrence in nonallergens, outperformed the FAO/WHO allergenicity rules [116]. Furthermore, as Table 6 shows, the motif-based allergenicity prediction scheme based on wavelet transform found areas of the allergenic tropomyosins that were not present in the nonallergenic tropomyosins. Further development of this method, taking into account the physicochemical properties of the amino acids and solvent accessibility, was able to correctly classify 93.0% of 229 allergens tested, and 99.95% of nonallergenic tropomyosins proteins [117].

Sequence similarity ranking in the Structural Database of Allergenic Proteins: the property distance scale PD

The FASTA search in SDAP is a rapid way to determine the overall similarity of large proteins. However, this program was not designed to compare short sequences, such as the linear IgE epitopes that have been identified by peptide mapping for many allergens [13,39,42,118]. Two different tools were incorporated in SDAP to look for short sequences in other known allergens: an exact search that finds short sequences identical to that of a known epitope, and a second tool to determine sequences that are close to the IgE epitope in property space. The *PD* tool determines similar sequences in other allergen entries in SDAP that have similar overall PCPs [72,73]. Peptides with identical sequences have a *PD* value of 0, and peptides with conservative substitutions of a few amino acids have a small *PD* value, typically in the range of 0 to 3. Peptides with a recognizable similarity in their physical chemical properties tend to have *PD* values lower than 10, whereas unrelated peptides have *PD* values that are much higher [119]. Table 7 shows two typical *PD* searches, performed with the automatic tools in SDAP, starting with the sequence of two IgE epitopes of the Jun a 3 protein.

Additional data are needed to determine the statistical significance of the identified regions in the other allergens, particularly in a database as large as SDAP. The *PD* search is designed to compare protein regions with lengths comparable with those of published linear IgE epitopes. Significance levels for the sequence-similarity index *PD* are set high enough to detect all peptides that are similar to an IgE epitope, but low enough to discriminate them from other regions in the ensemble of allergenic proteins that would match randomly. For the search, each area of all the sequences is individually matched, with a window for the sequence segment that moves progressively by one position. Thus a 200-amino-acid protein would have 194 different sequence windows of 7 amino acids, and 191 for a 10 mer. All *PD* searches in SDAP are followed by two histograms. The lowest-scoring window is determined for the best-matching peptide in the ~850 protein entries in SDAP. As the data in the heading of Table 7 indicate, for a *PD* search starting from a known epitope of Jun a 3, the average *PD* value for the best-scoring sequence window in each of the 854 full-length entries in SDAP was 12.15 (SD = 1.29). According to this test, values less than approximately 9 (mean value − 2 × the standard deviation) would be significantly similar to the test peptide. However, many similar sequences and isoforms are found in SDAP, which tends to skew the statistics for peptides. As a better estimate of what a random match would be, a second histogram summarizes the scores for all ~190,000 windows of a given size in all the

Table 7
Two typical *PD* searches, performed with the automatic tools in Structural Database of Allergen Proteins, starting with the sequence of two IgE epitopes of the Jun a 3 protein

No	Allergen	Source	*PD* Sequence similarity index	z(*PD*, all)	Start residue	Matching region	End residue
SDAP Search starting from epitope 3 of Jun a 3							
1	Jun a 3	Juniper	0.00	8.3364	146	ADINAVCPSELK	157
2	Cup a 3	Cedar	0.00	8.3364	120	ADINAVCPSELK	131
3	Pru av 2	Cherry	1.66	7.5620	157	ANVNAVCPSELQ	168
4	Mal d 2	Apple	6.63	5.2499	158	ANVNKVCPAPLQ	169
5	Lyc e NP24	Tomato	7.10	5.0309	148	ANINGECPRALK	159
6	Cap a 1	Pepper	7.31	4.9363	121	ANINGECPGSLR	132
SDAP Search starting from epitope 4 of Jun a 3							
1	Jun a 3	Juniper	0.00	9.0000	158	VDGGCNSACNVFKT	171
2	Cup a 3	Cedar	1.29	8.3504	132	VDGGCNSACNVLQT	145
3	Lyc e NP24	Tomato	8.20	4.8843	160	VPGGCNNPCTTFGG	173
4	Cap a 1	Pepper	8.20	4.8843	133	VPGGCNNPCTTFGG	146
5	Hev b 3	Latex	8.55	4.7090	41	LKPGVDTIENVVKT	54

Sequences most closely related to epitope 3 of Jun a 3 from mountain cedar pollen by the *PD* search show other PR5 proteins from fruits (*top*), and that of epitope 4 shows another known IgE epitope from latex (*bottom*; bold sequence). The column lists the order of sequences found, starting from each epitope sequence, the allergen name and source, the *PD* index (the lower the number, the more significant the sequence match), the Z-score[a] (the higher the number, the more significant the match), and finally the matching sequence. Note that no epitopes have been published for any of the fruit proteins, and that sequence of the kiwi thaumatin–like protein Act c 2 is only of the first 29 amino acids. The average *PD* value for the best scoring sequence in the 854 full-length entries in SDAP was 12.15 (SD = 1.29); the average *PD* value for all 190,530 possible windows was 17.24 (SD = 1.78).

[a] Using the *PD* distribution, the score z(*PD*) for a given match is calculated as: $z(PD) = \frac{|PD_{min} - PD_{ave}|}{SD(PD)}$.

SDAP allergen sequences. The average values in this histogram range from 17 to 26, depending on peptides. For the second example of Table 7, the average *PD* value for all 190,530 possible windows was 17.24 (SD = 1.78). According to these statistics for a random match, peptides with *PD* values less than 10 would be clear outliers.

To provide a sense of the significance of the match, Z-scores (which indicate the quality of the match relative to the database random distribution) are calculated automatically along with the *PD* value. The lower the *PD* score, the more closely related the peptide sequences are, but high Z-scores indicate better significance for the match.

The *PD* searches from two Jun a 3 IgE epitopes (see Table 7) illustrate the usefulness of using the *PD* value to identify potential epitopes and potentially cross-reactive allergenic proteins. For both epitopes, areas of thaumatin proteins from other pollens and fruits have the lowest *PD* value, consistent with their overall similarity according to the FASTA search (see Table 2). Note that the order of the sequences in the two tables is a bit different. Although the IgE epitopes have not been identified for the fruit allergens, the Jun a 3 epitope 4 has a low *PD* value to a known IgE epitope of the latex allergen Hev b 3. The significance of this finding for cross-reactivity has not been determined. Other results with the peanut allergen epitopes [13] have identified epitopes with similar IgE reactivity and predicted structure for *PD* scores as high as 9.5 to 10.

The *PD* search is a computational way to define the sequence relationship among known IgE epitopes and other sequences in allergenic proteins. The correlation of PD values to meaningful IgE cross-reactivity, and eventually to clinically relevant ones, is ongoing. However, initial tests indicate that this is a rapid way to quantify local similarities in known allergens. The structure of epitopes and their location on the protein surface (solvent exposure) are other possible factors determining whether a given sequence will bind IgE [13]. The authors believe the most promising methodology is to compare not only the sequences but also the structures of areas before suggesting possible cross-reactivity, as described in the next section.

Combining sequence and structural information to improve prediction

Many questions about the nature of the IgE epitopes of allergens remain unanswered. For example, why some individuals show cross-reactivity to homologous proteins in peanuts and tree nuts, whereas others with strong allergies only react to one or another of the homologous proteins [120]. Although single amino acid differences may be important in individual reactivity, a three-dimensional view of the identified IgE-binding sites can provide missing information about the possible relationships between structure and sequence. If IgE-binding sequences of related proteins have similar properties, the proposed methods that combine *PD* values with structural clues will have predictive ability if properly calibrated.

Once similar sequences have been identified by *PD* values, the structural information in SDAP can be used to understand which parts of an allergen sequence are likely to be surface-exposed, and thus likely to form an IgE binding surface [13,24]. Determining which residues are on the surface of an allergen (and thus most likely to react with an antibody) can also be determined rapidly and automatically using a program developed by GETAREA (http://www.scsb.utmb.edu/cgi-bin/get_a_form.tcl). This program has also been incorporated at the site, where the data can be quickly accessed for SDAP allergens of known or modeled structure. SDAP allows direct access to the experimental structures (of 586 SDAP allergens, 45 have known PDB structures). The authors estimate that for more than 90% of allergens that have unknown experimental structure, reliable models can be made based on results from fold recognition servers, such as 3DPSSM (http://www.sbg.bio.ic.ac.uk/~3dpssm/).

This article has only discussed linear epitopes, which occur next to one another in the sequence of a protein. A three-dimensionally folded protein may have epitopes formed from several areas of the sequence. The ConSurf [121] method has been used to detect patches of residues common to many allergens on the surface of allergen structures for Ara t 8, Act c 1, Bet v 1, and Ves v 5 [122]. The findings have not yet been tested experimentally. A combined method that uses sequence similarity and comparison of three-dimensional models was used to identify potentially cross-reactive peanut–lupine proteins [123] and search for potential new latex allergens [124]. The PCPMer program contains methodology to map conserved residues on the surface of proteins for detecting common areas. These *stereophysicochemical variability plots* are useful for distinguishing functional areas of viruses [125] and can also be used to identify regions that might constitute IgE epitopes. Alternatively, the authors are developing methods to map peptides that bind IgE to surface areas of allergens of known structure.

Summary

Similarities in sequence and structure of allergenic proteins can account for cross-reactivities among allergen sources [5,15,29,126–129] that may complicate the management of patients who have severe allergies [76,127,130].

Proteins are classified as allergens based on their ability to trigger responses in patients. Allergens may just be more potent forms of other proteins with similar surface areas that may have been the true sensitizing antigens during development of the disease. Therefore, how similar proteins must be to known triggers to represent significant risk for cross-reactivity is unknown. This problem is further complicated by the fact that some potent allergens can be rendered nonallergenic by selected point mutations and highly similar proteins, such as the glycinins of soybean and peanut (62% identity), and can provoke different responses [59].

This article outlines computational methodology to identify cross-reacting proteins at the molecular level, using the databases of allergenic proteins and their structures. Recent identification of the sequence and structure of allergenic proteins from pollen and foods has revealed similarities that might offer a structural explanation for their allergenicity and cross-reactivity [7,18,23,29,31,126,131]. Some of the recently developed search software tools, such as those implemented in SDAP, can help clinicians and patients find structural and functional relationships among known allergens and identify potentially cross-reacting antigens.

Clearly available methods cannot, with 100% accuracy, discriminate between closely related proteins according to their allergenicity. Instead, they indicate that certain proteins may be cross-reactive. These predictions can certainly be useful in developing dietary guidelines for individual patients and in designing specific immunotherapy.

References

[1] Sampson HA. Food allergy. Part 2: diagnosis and management. J Allergy Clin Immunol 1999;103(6):981–9.

[2] Sampson HA. Food allergy. Part 1: immunopathogenesis and clinical disorders. J Allergy Clin Immunol 1999;103(5):717–28.

[3] Sampson H. Food allergy: when mucosal immunity goes wrong. J Allergy Clin Immunol 2005;115:139–41.

[4] Vanek-Krebitz M, Hoffmann-Sommergruber K, Machado MLD, et al. Cloning and sequencing of Mal-D-1, the major allergen from apple (Malus-Domestica), and its immunological relationship to Bet-V-1, the major birch pollen allergen. Biochem Biophys Res Commun 1995;214(2):538–51.

[5] Scheurer S, Son DY, Boehm M, et al. Cross-reactivity and epitope analysis of Pru a 1, the major cherry allergen. Mol Immunol 1999;36(3):155–67.

[6] Rabjohn P, Helm EM, Stanley JS, et al. Molecular cloning and epitope analysis of the peanut allergen Ara h 3. J Clin Invest 1999;103(4):535–42.

[7] Breiteneder H, Ebner C. Molecular and biochemical classification of plant-derived food allergens. J Allergy Clin Immunol 2000;106(1):27–36.

[8] Jenkins JA, Griffiths-Jones S, Shewry PR, et al. Structural relatedness of plant food allergens with specific reference to cross-reactive allergens: an *in silico* analysis. J Allergy Clin Immunol 2005;115(1):163–70.

[9] Ferreira F, Hawranek T, Gruber P, et al. Allergic cross-reactivity: from gene to the clinic. Allergy 2004;59(3):243–67.

[10] Mari A. Multiple pollen sensitization: a molecular approach to the diagnosis. Int Arch Allergy Immunol 2001;125(1):57–65.

[11] Burks AW, Shin D, Cockrell G, et al. Mapping and mutational analysis of the IgE-binding epitopes on Ara h 1, a legume vicilin protein and a major allergen in peanut hypersensitivity. Eur J Biochem 1997;245(2):334–9.

[12] Shin DS, Compadre CM, Maleki SJ, et al. Biochemical and structural analysis of the IgE binding sites on Ara h 1, an abundant and highly allergenic peanut protein. J Biol Chem 1998;273(22):13753–9.

[13] Schein CH, Ivanciuc O, Braun W. Common physical-chemical properties correlate with similar structure of the IgE epitopes of peanut allergens. J Agric Food Chem 2005; 53(22):8752–9.

[14] de Leon MP, Glaspole IN, Drew AC, et al. Immunological analysis of allergenic cross-reactivity between peanut and tree nuts. Clin Exp Allergy 2003;33(9):1273–80.

[15] Eigenmann PA, Burks AW, Bannon GA, et al. Identification of unique peanut and soy allergens in sera adsorbed with cross-reacting antibodies. J Allergy Clin Immunol 1996; 98(5):969–78.

[16] Lopez-Torrejon G, Salcedo G, Martin-Esteban M, et al. Len c 1, a major allergen and vicilin from lentil seeds: protein isolation and cDNA cloning. J Allergy Clin Immunol 2003;112(6):1208–15.

[17] Wensing M, Knulst AC, Piersma S, et al. Patients with anaphylaxis to pea can have peanut allergy caused by cross-reactive IgE to vicilin (Ara h 1). J Allergy Clin Immunol 2003; 111(2):420–4.

[18] Midoro-Horiuti T, Brooks EG, Goldblum RM. Pathogenesis-related proteins of plants as allergens. Ann Allergy Asthma Immunol 2001;87(4):261–71.

[19] Asensio T, Crespo JF, Sanchez-Monge R, et al. Novel plant pathogenesis-related protein family involved in food allergy. J Allergy Clin Immunol 2004;114(4):896–9.

[20] Hoffmann-Sommergruber K. Pathogenesis-related (PR)-proteins identified as allergens. Biochem Soc Trans 2002;30:930–5.

[21] Elbez M, Kevers C, Hamdi S, et al. The plant pathogenesis-related PR-10 proteins. Acta Bot Gallica 2002;149(4):415–44.

[22] Midoro-Horiuti T, Goldblum R, Kurosky A, et al. Isolation and characterization of the mountain cedar (Juniperus ashei) pollen major allergen, Jun a 1. J Allergy Clin Immunol 1999;104:608–12.
[23] Soman KV, Midoro-Horiuti T, Ferreon JC, et al. Homology modeling and characterization of IgE epitopes of mountain cedar allergen Jun a 3. Biophys J 2000;79(3): 1601–9.
[24] Ivanciuc O, Mathura V, Midoro-Horiuti T, et al. Detecting potential IgE-reactive sites on food proteins using a sequence and structure database, SDAP-Food. J Agric Food Chem 2003;51(16):4830–7.
[25] Mari A. Importance of databases in experimental and clinical allergology. Int Arch Allergy Immunol 2005;138(1):88–96.
[26] Midoro-Horiuti T, Goldblum RN, Kurosky A, et al. Molecular cloning of the mountain cedar (Juniperus ashei) pollen major allergen, Jun a 1. J Allergy Clin Immunol 1999; 104(3):613–7.
[27] Midoro-Horiuti T, Mathura VS, Schein CH, et al. Major linear IgE epitopes of mountain cedar pollen allergen Jun a 1 map to the pectate lyase catalytic site. Mol Immunol 2003; 40(8):555–62.
[28] Midoro-Horiuti T, Schein CH, Mathura V, et al. Structural basis for epitope sharing between group 1 allergens of cedar pollen. Mol Immunol 2006;43(6):509–18.
[29] Fedorov AA, Ball T, Mahoney NM, et al. The molecular basis for allergen cross-reactivity: crystal structure and IgE epitope mapping of birch pollen profilin. Structure 1997;5(1): 33–45.
[30] Ferreira F, Ebner C, Kramer B, et al. Modulation of IgE reactivity of allergens by site-directed mutagenesis: potential use of hypoallergenic variants for immunotherapy. FASEB J 1998;12(2):231–42.
[31] Spangfort MD, Mirza O, Holm J, et al. The structure of major birch pollen allergens: epitopes, reactivity and cross-reactivity. Allergy 1999;50:23–6.
[32] Petersen A, Schramm G, Schlaak M, et al. Post-translational modifications influence IgE reactivity. Clin Exp Allergy 1998;28(3):315–21.
[33] Schramm G, Bufe A, Petersen A, et al. Mapping of IgE-binding epitopes on the recombinant major group I allergen of velvet grass pollen, rHol 1 1. J Allergy Clin Immunol 1997; 99(6):781–7.
[34] Lalla C, Tamborini E, Longhi R, et al. Human recombinant antibody fragments specific for a rye-grass pollen allergen: characterization and potential applications. Mol Immunol 1996; 33:1049–58.
[35] Flicker S, Vrtala S, Steinberger P, et al. A human monoclonal IgE antibody defines a highly allergenic fragment of the major timothy grass pollen allergen, Phl p 5: molecular, immunological, and structural characterization of the epitope-containing domain. J Immunol 2000;165:3849–59.
[36] Wal JM. Bovine milk allergenicity. Ann Allergy Asthma Immunol 2004;93(5):S2–11.
[37] Natale M, Bisson C, Monti G, et al. Cow's milk allergens identification by two-dimensional immunoblotting and mass spectrometry. Mol Nutr Food Res 2004;48(5):363–9.
[38] Pourpak Z, Mostafaie A, Hasan Z, et al. A laboratory method for purification of major cow's milk allergens. J Immunoassay Immunochem 2004;25(4):385–97.
[39] Elsayed S, Hill DJ, Do TV. Evaluation of the allergenicity and antigenicity of bovine-milk alpha s1-casein using extensively purified synthetic peptides. Scand J Immunol 2004;60(5): 486–93.
[40] Cocco RR, Jarvinen KM, Sampson HA, et al. Mutational analysis of major, sequential IgE-binding epitopes in alpha(s1)-casein, a major cow's milk allergen. J Allergy Clin Immunol 2003;112(2):433–7.
[41] Ehn BM, Ekstrand B, Bengtsson U, et al. Modification of IgE binding during heat processing of the cow's milk allergen beta-lactoglobulin. J Agric Food Chem 2004;52(5): 1398–403.

[42] Jarvinen KM, Chatchatee P, Bardina L, et al. IgE and IgG binding epitopes on alpha-lactalbumin and beta-lactoglobulin in cow's milk allergy. Int Arch Allergy Immunol 2001; 126(2):111–8.
[43] Adel-Patient K, Creminon C, Boquet D, et al. Genetic immunisation with bovine beta-lactoglobulin cDNA induces a preventive and persistent inhibition of specific anti-BLG IgE response in mice. Int Arch Allergy Immunol 2001;126(1):59–67.
[44] Mine Y, Rupa P. Immunological and biochemical properties of egg allergens. Worlds Poult Sci J 2004;60(3):321–30.
[45] Mizumachi K, Kurisaki J. Localization of T cell epitope regions of chicken ovomucoid recognized by mice. Biosci Biotechnol Biochem 2003;67(4):712–9.
[46] Mine Y, Sasaki E, Zhang JW. Reduction of antigenicity and allergenicity of genetically modified egg white allergen, ovomucoid third domain. Biochem Biophys Res Commun 2003;302(1):133–7.
[47] Mine Y, Zhang JW. Identification and fine mapping of IgG and IgE epitopes in ovomucoid. Biochem Biophys Res Commun 2002;292(4):1070–4.
[48] Fremont S, Kanny G, Nicolas JP, et al. Prevalence of lysozyme sensitization in an egg-allergic population. Allergy 1997;52(2):224–8.
[49] Ayuso R, Lehrer SB, Reese G. Identification of continuous, allergenic regions of the major shrimp allergen Pen a 1 (tropomyosin). Int Arch Allergy Immunol 2002;127(1):27–37.
[50] Reese G, Ayuso R, Leong-Kee SM, et al. Epitope mapping and mutational substitution analysis of the major shrimp allergen Pen a 1 (tropomyosin). J Allergy Clin Immunol 2002;109(1):S307.
[51] Samson KTR, Chen FH, Miura K, et al. IgE binding to raw and boiled shrimp proteins in atopic and nonatopic patients with adverse reactions to shrimp. Int Arch Allergy Immunol 2004;133(3):225–32.
[52] Van Do T, Hordvik I, Endresen C, et al. Characterization of parvalbumin, the major allergen in Alaska pollack, and comparison with codfish Allergen M. Mol Immunol 2005;42(3):345–53.
[53] Swoboda I, Bugajska-Schretter A, Verdino P, et al. Recombinant carp parvalbumin, the major cross-reactive fish allergen: a tool for diagnosis and therapy of fish allergy. Allergy 2002;57:80.
[54] Swoboda I, Bugajska-Schretter A, Valenta R, et al. Recombinant fish parvalbumins: candidates for diagnosis and treatment of fish allergy. Allergy 2002;57:94–6.
[55] Moreno FJ, Maldonado BM, Wellner N, et al. Thermostability and in vitro digestibility of a purified major allergen 2S albumin (Ses i 1) from white sesame seeds (Sesamum indicum L.). Biochim Biophys Acta 2005;1752(2):142–53.
[56] Robotham JM, Wang F, Seamon V, et al. Ana o 3, an important cashew nut (Anacardium occidentale L.) allergen of the 2S albumin family. J Allergy Clin Immunol 2005;115(6): 1284–90.
[57] Palomares O, Cuesta-Herranz J, Rodriiguez R, et al. A recombinant precursor of the mustard allergen Sin a 1 retains the biochemical and immunological features of the heterodimeric native protein. Int Arch Allergy Immunol 2005;137(1):18–26.
[58] Moreno FJ, Mellon FA, Wickham MSJ, et al. Stability of the major allergen Brazil nut 2S albumin (Ber e 1) to physiologically relevant in vitro gastrointestinal digestion. FEBS J 2005;272(2):341–52.
[59] Beardslee TA, Zeece MG, Sarath G, et al. Soybean glycinin G1 acidic chain shares IgE epitopes with peanut allergen Ara h 3. Int Arch Allergy Immunol 2000;123(4): 299–307.
[60] Helm RM, Cockrell G, Connaughton C, et al. A soybean G2 glycinin allergen-1. Identification and characterization. Int Arch Allergy Immunol 2000;123(3):205–12.
[61] Rabjohn P, Burks AW, Sampson HA, et al. Mutational analysis of the IgE-binding epitopes of the peanut allergen, Ara h 3: a member of the glycinin family of seed-storage proteins. J Allergy Clin Immunol 1999;103(1):S101.

[62] Bolhaar S, van Ree R, Bruijnzeel-Koomen C, et al. Allergy to jackfruit: a novel example of Bet v 1-related food allergy. Allergy. 2004;59(11):1187–92.
[63] Bolhaar S, van Ree R, Ma Y, et al. Severe allergy to sharon fruit caused by birch pollen. Int Arch Allergy Immunol 2005;136(1):45–52.
[64] Bolhaar S, Zuidmeer L, Ma Y, et al. A mutant of the major apple allergen, Mal d 1, demonstrating hypo-allergenicity in the target organ by double-blind placebo-controlled food challenge. Clin Exp Allergy 2005;35(12):1638–44.
[65] Bucher X, Pichler WJ, Dahinden CA, et al. Effect of tree pollen specific, subcutaneous immunotherapy on the oral allergy syndrome to apple and hazelnut. Allergy 2004;59(12): 1272–6.
[66] Mari A, Ballmer-Weber BK, Vieths S. The oral allergy syndrome: improved diagnostic and treatment methods. Curr Opin Allergy Clin Immunol 2005;5(3):267–73.
[67] Bolhaar S, Tiemessen MM, Zuidmeer L, et al. Efficacy of birch-pollen immunotherapy on cross-reactive food allergy confirmed by skin tests and double-blind food challenges. Clin Exp Allergy 2004;34(5):761–9.
[68] Gendel SM. Bioinformatics and food allergens. J AOAC Int 2004;87:1417–22.
[69] Glaspole IN, de Leon MP, Rolland JM, et al. Characterization of the T-cell epitopes of a major peanut allergen, Ara h 2. Allergy 2005;60:35–40.
[70] Breiteneder H, Mills ENC. Molecular properties of food allergens. J Allergy Clin Immunol 2005;115:14–23.
[71] Brusic V, Millot M, Petrovsky N, et al. Allergen databases. Allergy 2003;58(11):1093–100.
[72] Ivanciuc O, Schein CH, Braun W. SDAP: database and computational tools for allergenic proteins. Nucleic Acids Res 2003;31(1):359–62.
[73] Ivanciuc O, Schein CH, Braun W. Data mining of sequences and 3D structures of allergenic proteins. Bioinformatics 2002;18(10):1358–64.
[74] Schein CH, Ivanciuc O, Braun W. Structural database of allergenic proteins (SDAP). In: Maleki SJ, Burks AW, Helm RM, editors. Food allergy. Washington, DC: ASM Press; 2006. p. 257–83.
[75] Stadler MB, Stadler BM. Allergenicity prediction by protein sequence. FASEB Journal 2003;17(6):1141–3.
[76] WHO. Evaluation of allergenicity of genetically modified foods. Report of a joint FAO/WHO expert consultation. Geneva (Switzerland): World Health Organization; 2001.
[77] WHO. Joint FAO/WHO food standards programme. Codex Ad Hoc intergovernmental task force on foods derived from biotechnology. Yokohama (Japan): World Health Organization; 2003. Available at: http://www.codexalimentarius.net/. Accessed September 18, 2006.
[78] Pearson W. Rapid and sensitive sequence comparison with FASTP and FASTA. Methods Enzymol 1990;183:63–98.
[79] Conte LL, Ailey B, Hubbard TJP, et al. SCOP: a structural classification of proteins database. Nucleic Acids Res 2000;28(1):257–9.
[80] Gilbert D, Westhead D, Nagano N, et al. Motif-based searching in TOPS protein topology databases. Bioinformatics 1999;15(4):317–26.
[81] Pearl FMG, Martin N, Bray JE, et al. A rapid classification protocol for the CATH Domain Database to support structural genomics. Nucleic Acids Res 2001;29(1): 223–7.
[82] Shindyalov IN, Bourne PE. Protein structure alignment by incremental combinatorial extension (CE) of the optimal path. Protein Eng 1998;11(9):739–47.
[83] Holm L, Sander C. Mapping the protein universe. Science 1996;273:595–602.
[84] Gibrat JF, Madej T, Bryant SH. Surprising similarities in structure comparison. Curr Opin Struct Biol 1996;6(3):377–85.
[85] Rabjohn P, West C, Connaughton C, et al. Modification of peanut allergen Ara h 3: effects on IgE binding and T cell stimulation. Int Arch Allergy Immunol 2002;128:15–23.

[86] Bannon G, Cockrell G, Connaughton C, et al. Engineering, characterization and in vitro efficacy of the major peanut allergens for use in immunotherapy. Int Arch Allergy Immunol 2001;124:70–2.

[87] Li XM, Srivastava K, Huleatt JW, et al. Engineered recombinant peanut protein and heat-killed Listeria monocytogenes coadministration protects against peanut-induced anaphylaxis in a murine model. J Immunol 2003;170:3289–95.

[88] vanRee R, Antonicelli L, Akkerdaas JH, et al. Possible induction of food allergy during mite immunotherapy. Allergy 1996;51(2):108–13.

[89] Breiteneder H, Mills ENC. Plant food allergens—structural and functional aspects of allergenicity. Biotechnol Adv 2005;23(6):395–9.

[90] Schein CH. The shape of the messenger: using protein structural information to design novel cytokine-based therapeutics. Curr Pharm Des 2002;8(24):213–30.

[91] Weber RW. Patterns of pollen cross-reactivity. J Allergy Clin Immunol 2003;112: 229–39.

[92] Breiteneder H, Radauer C. A classification of plant food allergens. J Allergy Clin Immunol 2004;113(5):821–30.

[93] Hartl A, Kiesslich J, Weiss R, et al. Isoforms of the major allergen of birch pollen induce different immune responses after genetic immunization. Int Arch Allergy Immunol 1999; 120(1):17–29.

[94] Ferreira F, Hirthenlehner K, Briza P, et al. Isoforms of atopic allergens with reduced allergenicity but conserved T cell antigenicity: possible use for specific immunotherapy. Int Arch Allergy Immunol 1997;113(1–3):125–7.

[95] Ferreira F, Hirtenlehner K, Jilek A, et al. Dissection of immunoglobulin E and T lymphocyte reactivity of isoforms of the major birch pollen allergen Bet v 1: potential use of hypoallergenic isoforms for immunotherapy. J Exp Med 1996;183(2): 599–609.

[96] Thomas K, Bannon G, Hefle S, et al. In silico methods for evaluating human allergenicity to novel proteins: International Bioinformatics Workshop Meeting Report, 23-24 February 2005. Toxicol Sci 2005;88(2):307–10.

[97] Aalberse RC, Stadler BM. In silico predictability of allergenicity: from amino acid sequence via 3-D structure to allergenicity. Mol Nutr Food Res 2006;50(7):625–7.

[98] Riaz T, Hor HL, Krishnan A, et al. WebAllergen: a web server for predicting allergenic proteins. Bioinformatics 2005;21(10):2570–1.

[99] Li KB, Issac P, Krishnan A. Predicting allergenic proteins using wavelet transform. Bioinformatics 2004;20(16):2572–8.

[100] Saha S, Raghava GPS. AlgPred: prediction of allergenic proteins and mapping of IgE epitopes. Nucleic Acids Res 2006;34:W202–9.

[101] Fiers M, Kleter GA, Nijland H, et al. Allermatch (TM), a webtool for the prediction of potential allergenicity according to current FAO/WHO Codex alimentarius guidelines. BMC Bioinformatics 2004;5:133.

[102] Brusic V, Petrovsky N. Bioinformatics for characterisation of allergens, allergenicity and allergic crossreactivity. Trends Immunol 2003;24(5):225–8.

[103] Hileman RE, Silvanovich A, Goodman RE, et al. Bioinformatic methods for allergenicity assessment using a comprehensive allergen database. Int Arch Allergy Immunol 2002; 128(4):280–91.

[104] Bindsley-Jensen C, Sten E, Earl LK, et al. Assessment of the potential allergenicity of ice structuring protein type III HPLC 12 using the FAO/WHO 2001 decision tree for novel foods. Food Chem Toxicol 2003;41(1):81–7.

[105] Baderschneider B, Crevel RWR, Earl LK, et al. Sequence analysis and resistance to pepsin hydrolysis as part of an assessment of the potential allergenicity of ice structuring protein type III HPLC 12. Food Chem Toxicol 2002;40(7):965–78.

[106] Singh AK, Mehta AK, Sridhara S, et al. Allergenicity assessment of transgenic mustard (Brassica juncea) expressing bacterial codA gene. Allergy 2006;61(4):491–7.

[107] Soeria-Atmadja D, Zorzet A, Gustafsson MG, et al. Statistical evaluation of local alignment features predicting allergenicity using supervised classification algorithms. Int Arch Allergy Immunol 2004;133(2):101–12.

[108] Soeria-Atmadja D, Wallman M, Björklund ÅK, et al. External cross-validation for unbiased evaluation of protein family detectors: application to allergens. Proteins 2005;61(4): 918–25.

[109] Zorzet A, Gustafsson M, Hammerling U. Prediction of food protein allergenicity: a bioinformatic learning systems approach. In Silico Biol 2004;2:525–34.

[110] Mills EN, Jenkins J, Marigheto N, et al. Allergens of the cupin superfamily. Biochem Soc Trans 2002;30(6):925–9.

[111] Venkatarajan MS, Braun W. New quantitative descriptors of amino acids based on multidimensional scaling of a large number of physical-chemical properties. J Mol Model 2001; 7(12):445–53.

[112] Mathura VS, Schein CH, Braun W. Identifying property based sequence motifs in protein families and superfamilies: application to DNase I related endonucleases. Bioinformatics 2003;19(11):1381–90.

[113] Kleter GA, Peijnenburg A. Presence of potential allergy-related linear epitopes in novel proteins from conventional crops and the implication for the safety assessment of these crops with respect to the current testing of genetically modified crops. Plant Biotechnol J 2003;1(5):371–80.

[114] Saha S, Raghava GPS. Prediction of continuous B-cell epitopes in an antigen using recurrent neural network. Proteins 2006;65:40–8.

[115] Silvanovich A, Nemeth MA, Song P, et al. The value of short amino acid sequence matches for prediction of protein allergenicity. Toxicol Sci 2006;90(1):252–8.

[116] Björklund ÅK, Soeria-Atmadja D, Zorzet A, et al. Supervised identification of allergen-representative peptides for in silico detection of potentially allergenic proteins. Bioinformatics 2005;21(1):39–50.

[117] Cui J, Han LY, Li H, et al. Computer prediction of allergen proteins from sequence-derived protein structural and physicochemical properties. Mol Immunol 2007;44(4):514–20.

[118] Shreffler WG, Beyer K, Chu TH, et al. Microarray immunoassay: association of clinical history, in vitro IgE function, and heterogeneity of allergenic peanut epitopes. J Allergy Clin Immunol 2004;113(4):776–82.

[119] Ivanciuc O, Oezguen N, Mathura V, et al. Using property based sequence motifs and 3D modeling to determine structure and functional regions in CASP5 targets. Curr Med Chem 2004;11(5):583–93.

[120] Teuber SS, Beyer K. Peanut, tree nut and seed allergies. Curr Opin Allergy Clin Immunol 2004;4(3):201–3.

[121] Glaser F, Pupko T, Paz I, et al. ConSurf: identification of functional regions in proteins by surface-mapping of phylogenetic information. Bioinformatics 2003;19(1):163–4.

[122] Furmonaviciene R, Sutton BJ, Glaser F, et al. An attempt to define allergen-specific molecular surface features: a bioinformatic approach. Bioinformatics 2005;21(23):4201–4.

[123] Guarneri F, Guarneri C, Benvenga S. Identification of potentially cross-reactive peanut-lupine proteins by computer-assisted search for amino acid sequence homology. Int Arch Allergy Immunol 2005;138(4):273–7.

[124] Guarneri F, Guarneri C, Guarneri B, et al. In silico identification of potential new latex allergens. Clin Exp Allergy 2006;36(7):916–9.

[125] Schein CH, Zhou B, Braun W. Stereophysicochemical variability plots highlight conserved antigenic areas in Flaviviruses. Virol J 2005;2:40.

[126] Ipsen H, Lowenstein H. Basic features of cross-reactivity in tree and grass pollen allergy. Clin Rev Allergy Immunol 1997;15(4):389–96.

[127] Lehrer SI, Ayuso R, Reese G. Current understanding of food allergens. In: Fu TJ, Gendel SM, editors. Genetically engineered foods: assessing potential allergenicity, vol. 964. New York: The New York Academy of Sciences; 2002. p. 69–85.

[128] Leung PSC, Chow WK, Duffey S, et al. IgE reactivity against a cross-reactive allergen in crustacea and mollusca: evidence fev tropomyosin as the common allergen. J Allergy Clin Immunol 1996;98(5):954–61.
[129] Sparholt SH, Larsen JN, Ipsen H, et al. Crossreactivity and T-cell epitope specificity of Bet v 1-specific T cells suggest the involvement of multiple isoallergens in sensitization to birch pollen. Clin Exp Allergy 1997;27(8):932–41.
[130] Bousquet J, Knani J, Hejjaoui A, et al. Heterogeneity of atopy. 1. Clinical and immunological characteristics of patients allergic to cypress pollen. Allergy 1993;48(3):183–8.
[131] Aalberse RC. Structural biology of allergens. J Allergy Clin Immunol 2000;106(2): 228–38.

ELSEVIER
SAUNDERS

Immunol Allergy Clin N Am
27 (2007) 29–44

IMMUNOLOGY
AND ALLERGY
CLINICS
OF NORTH AMERICA

Calcium-Binding Proteins and Their Role in Allergic Diseases

Nicole Wopfner, PhD[a,*], Oliver Dissertori, BSc[b], Fatima Ferreira, PhD[a], Peter Lackner, PhD[b,*]

[a] *Department of Molecular Biology, Christian Doppler Laboratory for Allergy Diagnostic and Therapy, University of Salzburg, Hellbrunnerstrasse 34, A-5020 Salzburg, Austria*
[b] *Department of Molecular Biology, Division of Genomics, University of Salzburg, Hellbrunnerstrasse 34, A-5020 Salzburg, Austria*

Extensive cross-reactivity within allergenic plants likely is caused by three families of widely distributed panallergens: the profilins, the calcium-binding proteins (CBPs), and the nonspecific lipid transfer proteins.

Various CBPs have been isolated from pollen (grasses, trees, and weeds), parasites, fish, and man and were described as highly cross-reactive allergens not just in pollen but also in food [1].

CBPs exhibit a great diversity of composition, structure, Ca^{2+}-binding, and target interaction properties [2]. These proteins may act simply as calcium carrier and buffer, or—because of calcium-induced changes—interact with proteins in a calcium-dependent manner, and, thus, act as cellular messengers [3]. In general, calcium-binding proteins can be classified into 32 distinct subfamilies of proteins that may contain from two to eight calcium-binding domains called EF-hands (helix-loop-helix motifs). The EF-hand superfamily of proteins includes proteins like calmodulin, troponin C, myosin light chain, and more than 100 others. The canonical EF-hand is a highly conserved portion of these proteins and consists of an alpha helix, a loop around the bound calcium ion, and a second alpha helix (Fig. 1). Calcium ions usually bind to the EF-hand domain through four carboxylate or carboxyamide groups and one single backbone carbonyl oxygen placed in the loop with a specific spacing [4]. There are more than 3000 EF-hand–related entries in the National Center for Biotechnology Information

This work was supported by Project S-8802 from the Austrian Research Council (FWF).
* Corresponding author.
E-mail addresses: nicole.wopfner@sbg.ac.at (N. Wopfner); peter.lackner@sbg.ac.at (P. Lackner).

0889-8561/07/$ - see front matter
doi:10.1016/j.iac.2006.10.003 ***immunology.theclinics.com***

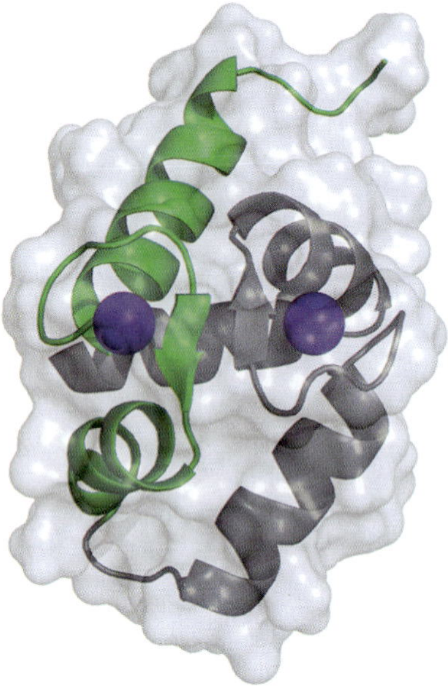

Fig. 1. Structure of the monomeric Bet v 4 protein. The molecule consists of two similar structural subunits in a symmetric arrangement. A single EF-hand is highlighted in green, calcium ions are in dark blue. This figure was prepared with PyMOL (DeLano WL, The PyMOL Molecular Graphics System, 2002, http://www.pymol.org).

Reference Sequence Data bank, but just a small number of the EF-hand superfamily was described as allergens. The official list of allergens maintained by the International Union of Immunological Societies Allergen Nomenclature Subcommittee (www.allergen.org; version February 20, 2006) features 16 calcium-binding allergens: 10 from pollen and 6 from animal sources. The allergome database (www.allergome.org; data retrieved on August 21, 2006) lists 64 calcium-binding allergens: 34 from pollen and 30 from animal sources.

Calcium-binding proteins as allergens

More than 30 years ago, parvalbumin, a major fish allergen, was the first described and characterized calcium-binding allergen [5,6]. Since then, a great number of pollen and food allergens was reported, and sequence analysis of allergen-encoding cDNAs revealed the presence of the typical calcium-binding EF-hand motifs within many of the cloned allergens.

Therefore, calcium-binding allergens also may be grouped according to immunologic cross-reactivity and not only according to the number of EF-hand domains. Table 1 gives an overview of the calcium-binding allergens, grouped according to the allergen source. The two major cross-reactive allergen families include the EF-hand pollen allergens from trees,

Table 1
Calcium-binding allergens from pollen, food, and animals

Pollen allergens (Polcalcins)	Tree	Grass	Weed
	Aln g 4	Agr c	Amb a 9
	Bet v 3	Ant o	Amb a 10
	Bet v 4[a]	Ave s	Art v 5
	Car b	Bro i	Bra n 1
	Fra e 3	Cyn d 7	Bra n 2
	Jun o 4	Dac g	Bra r 1
	Ole e 3	Dis s	Bra r 2
	Ole e 8	Fes e	Che a 3[a]
	Pho d	Lol p	Par j
	Que a	Phl p 7[a]	
	Rob p	Poa p	
	Syr v 3	Sor h	
		Tri a	
		Zea m	
Food allergens (Parvalbumins)	Fish	Amphibian	
	Bar s	Ran e 1	
	Cyp c 1.01	Ran e 2	
	Cyp c 1.02		
	Gad c 1		
	Gad m 1		
	Sal s 1		
	Sco a 1		
	Sco j 1		
	Sco s 1		
	Sti 1		
	The c 1		
Animals	Arthropods	Mammalian	
	Bla g 6	Bos d 3	
	Der f 17	Hom s 4	

Calcium-binding allergens containing 2 EF-hand motifs are listed. Calcium-binding allergens with 3 EF-hands are underlined and with 4 EF-hands are in bold.

Abbreviations: Agr c, *Agropyron cristatum* (Quack grass); Alg n, *Alnus glutinosa* (Alder); Amba, *Ambrosia artemisiifolia* (Ragweed); Ant o, *Anthoxanthum odoratum*, (Sweet vernal grass); Art v, *Artemisia vulgaris* (Mugwort); Ave s, *Avena sativa* (Cultivated oat); Bar s, *Boreogadus saida* (Arctic cod); Bet v, *Betula verrucosa* (Birch); Bla g, *Blattella germanica* (German cockroach); Bos d, *Bos domesticus* (Cattle); Bra n, *Brassica napus* (Rapeseed); Bra r, *Brassica rapa* (Turnip); Bro i, *Bromus inermis* (Smooth brome grass); Car b, *Carbinus betulus* (Hornbeam); Che a, *Chenopodium album* (Goosefoot); Cyn d, *Cynodon dactylon* (Bermuda grass); Cyp c, *Cyprinus carpio* (Carp); Dac g, *Dactylis glomerata* (Orchard grass); Der f, *Dermatophagoides farinae* (House dust mite); Dis s, *Distichlis stricta* (Salt grass); Fes e, *Festuca elatior* (Reed fescue); Fra e, *Fraxinus excelsior* (Ash); Gad c, *Gadus callarias* (Codfish); Gad m, *Gadus morhua* (Atlantic cod); Hom s, *Homo sapiens* (Human); Jun o, *Juniperus oxycedrus* (Prickly juniper); Lol p, *Lolium perenne* (Rye grass); Ole e, *Olea europaea* (Olive); Par j, *Parietaria judaica* (Pellitory); Phl p, *Phleum pratense* (Timothy grass); Phl d, *Phoenix dactylifera* (Date palm tree); Poa p, *Poa pratensis* (Kentucky blue grass); Que a, *Quercus alba* (White oak); Ran e, *Rana esculenta* (Edible frog); Rob p, *Robinia pseudoacacia* (Locust tree); Sal s, *Salmon salar* (Atlantic salmon); Sco a, *Scomber australasicus* (Pacific mackerel); Sco j, *Scomber japonicus* (Spotted mackerel); Sco s, *Scomber scombrus* (Atlantic mackerel); Sor h, *Sorghum halepense* (Johnson grass); Sti l, *Stizostedion lucioperca* (Perch); Syr v, *Syringa vulgaris* (Common lilac); The c, *Theragra chalcogramma* (Alaska pollock); Tri a, *Triticum aestivum* (Wheat); Zea m, *Zea mays* (Maize).

[a] Allergens with known three-dimensional structure.

grasses, and weeds and the parvalbumins from various fish species (carp, cod, mackerel, and salmon). Pollen calcium-binding allergens (polcalcins) can be classified into three groups according to the number of EF-hands contained in their sequence. Calcium-binding allergens containing 2EF-hands have been detected and characterized in birch (Bet v 4), timothy grass (Phl p 7), Bermuda grass (Cyn d 7), alder (Aln g 4), olive tree (Ole e 3), goosefoot (Che a 3), ragweed (Amb a 9), mugwort (Art v 5), lilac (Syr v 3), rape seed (Bra n 1, Bra n 2, Bra r 1, and Bra r 2), and some other trees and grasses [7–16]. CBPs with 3EF-hand domains were described in birch (Bet v 3) [17] and ragweed (Amb a 10) [7], and those with 4EF-hands were described in olive pollen (Ole e 8) [18] and prickly juniper (Jun o 4) [19].

Parvalbumins, the dominating fish allergen, were described in fish species like carp, tuna, cod, mackerel, perch, Alaska pollock, and salmon. Fish parvalbumin is a stable CBP; exposure to extremes in pH and temperature does not alter its IgE reactivity [20].

A human CBP, Hom s 4, recognized by IgE autoantibodies from patients who had atopic dermatitis, was described recently [21]. Hom s 4 is a 54-kd basic protein containing two typical calcium-binding domains separated by an unusually long alpha-helical domain; thus, it constitutes a novel subfamily of CBPs. Hom s 4–homologous proteins were found by sequence comparison in mice, fruit flies, and nematodes. The protein is strongly expressed in epidermal keratinocytes and dermal endothelial cells. Hom s 4 induced T helper 1-biased immune responses, which were accompanied by the release of interferon (IFN)-γ. Hom s 4–induced IFN-γ production was found in normal individuals, in patients who had chronic inflammatory skin diseases, and in T helper 2-prone atopic persons [21]. Therefore, Hom s 4 might contribute to chronic skin inflammation in atopic as well as in nonatopic individuals.

Possible physiologic role of allergenic calcium-binding proteins

Most CBPs are expressed preferentially in certain tissues. The expression pattern of plant-derived CBPs was investigated by Northern blot analysis of calcium-binding allergens from *Brassica* pollen; this demonstrated that these proteins were preferentially expressed in anthers at the later developmental stage and in mature pollen [16]. Northern blot analysis of CBPs from Bermuda grass, timothy grass, mugwort, birch (Bet v 3 and Bet v 4), and olive confirmed that the expression of these CBPs is restricted to pollen [9,10,15,17]. Because CBPs are tightly involved in the distribution and control of the intracellular calcium levels in plants, it is speculated that these allergenic CBPs might play a role in pollen germination, a process known to be critically dependent on the presence of calcium ions [22]. In this respect, a possible biologic role of 2EF-hand CBPs in pollen germination and tube growth was investigated using lily pollen as model system [10]. When recombinant Bet v 4 was introduced into growing lily pollen tubes by iontophoresis, cytoplasmic streaming stopped in the vicinity of the electrode tip, and a slight depolarization of the membrane voltage could be measured. These effects were not observed with Ca^{2+}-binding–deficient mutants of Bet v 4. Thus, Bet v 4, and, possibly, homologous proteins with 2EF-hand domains, represents a new class of pollen-specific Ca^{2+}-binding allergens that may have a physiologic role as inhibitors of cytoplasmic streaming in outgrowing pollen tubes [10].

Parvalbumin is a low molecular weight (9–11 kd) protein in muscle from fish and amphibians that aids in relaxation from contraction. Parvalbumin binds myoplasmic Ca^{2+} during muscle contractions, reducing calcium concentration and enhancing muscle relaxation. Each molecule of parvalbumin has two binding sites, and these sites have high affinity for Ca^{2+} and moderate affinity for Mg^{2+}. Parvalbumin binds Ca^{2+} with a higher affinity than troponin C, but less affinity than the sarcoplasmic reticulum Ca^{2+} ATPase pumps. As Ca^{2+} is pumped back into the sarcoplasmic reticulum by Ca^{2+}-ATPase pumps and the myoplasmic $[Ca^{2+}]$ decreases, parvalbumin competes with troponin C to bind to the sarcoplasmic Ca^{2+}, accelerating the relaxation of muscle. There is a wide range in the total parvalbumin content of fish muscle, which, in turn, affects relaxation. Typically, greater parvalbumin content is associated with fast-twitch muscle of various vertebrates with high rates of relaxation [23].

Calcium-binding allergens from pollen (polcalcins)

In a recent review [24], pollen allergen sequences were analyzed with respect to protein family membership, taxonomic distribution of protein families, and interspecies variability. Pollen allergens were classified into 29 of 7868 protein families in the Pfam database release 4.2 (http://www.sanger.ac.uk/Software/Pfam/). Expansins, profilins, and CBPs constitute the major families of pollen allergens. All calcium-binding allergens from pollen show low sequence similarities (39%–42%) to calmodulins and calmodulin-like proteins from vegetative plant tissue and from animals, suggesting that they might constitute a distinct subfamily of CBPs.

At least three types of allergenic EF-hand CBPs are expressed in pollen tissue: a ubiquitous family of CBPs with 2EF-hand domains, calcium-binding allergens with 3EF-hand motifs, and the 4EF-hand CBPs.

2EF-hand calcium-binding allergens

Calcium-binding allergens described so far are low molecular weight (8–25 kd), mostly acidic proteins that are released rapidly after hydration of the pollen. The major family of the pollen CBPs is represented by the 2EF-hand domain allergens with molecular weights between 8 and 9 kd. The best characterized are Bet v 4 and Alg n 4 from trees, Cyn d 7 and Phl p 7 from grasses, and the weed CBPs: Bra n 1, Bra n 2, Bra r 1, and Bra r 2.

The authors identified a ragweed polcalcin designated Amb a 9 (GenBank Accession AY894657) by screening a cDNA library with patients' IgE [25]. A 2EF-hand allergen also was present in mugwort pollen extracts by IgG immunoblots using rabbit anti–Phl p 7 sera [26]. In the authors' laboratory, a cDNA clone coding for mugwort polcalcin (GenBank Accession AY904434) was isolated and designated Art v 5 (N. Wopfner, PhD, unpublished data, 2007). Amb a 9 and Art v 5 show sequence homology to birch Bet v 4. Approximately 10% to 30% of patients who were allergic to weed pollen displayed IgE reactivity to Amb a 9 and Art v 5 [7].

Within the group of 2EF-hand calcium-binding pollen allergens, amino acid sequence comparison revealed significant sequence similarity (60%–80%) and strict conservation of the amino acid residues involved in calcium binding. The prevalence of IgE reactivity to this subfamily of proteins ranged from 5% to 46% for Bet v 4 and Che a 3, respectively [10,13]; 20% to 35% for Ole e 3, Art v 5, Amb a 9, and Amb a 10 [7,9,27]; and 10% for Phl p 7 [13]. The prevalence of IgE reactivity for each allergen seems to depend on the geographical area of the tested patients. When Moverare and colleagues [28] compared different European populations' reactivity to Bet v 4, prevalence values between 5% and 11% for patients from North and Central Europe, and 27% for Italian patients were observed.

Three EF-hand calcium-binding proteins

So far, the only members of the 3EF-hand calcium-binding allergen subfamily are Bet v 3 from birch [17] and Amb a 10 from ragweed [7]. Different from the 2EF-hand CBPs, IgE binding to Bet v 3 absolutely required protein-bound Ca^{2+}, and depletion with EGTA led to a reversible loss of IgE binding [17].

Four EF-hand calcium-binding proteins

Two calcium-binding proteins with 4EF-hand motifs were described: Ole e 8 [18,29] from olive pollen and Jun o 4 (formerly Jun o 2) from prickly juniper [19]. The presence of cross-reactive epitopes in recombinant (r) Jun o 4 and in pollen extracts from taxonomically related and unrelated species (eg, mountain cedar, cypress, common cypress, rye grass, *Parietaria*, and olive) was demonstrated by IgE immunoblotting experiments [19]. Similar to Bet v 3, depletion of calcium led to a loss of IgE-binding activity. Although Ole e 8 and Jun o 4 contain 4EF-hand calcium-binding domains, they show overall low sequence identity.

Parvalbumins: cross-reactive calcium-binding food allergens

Parvalbumins are major food allergens that are abundant in muscle from fish and amphibians. Especially in countries where most of the population works in the fishing industry and where fish is a staple food, parvalbumins are one of the most important causes of IgE-mediated food hypersensitivity. In a Norwegian study, it was estimated that 1 in 1000 individuals was allergic to fish [30].

Parvalbumins are CBPs of low molecular weight (10-12 kd) that are resistant to heat, chemical denaturation, and proteolytic enzymes [31,32]. Initially, parvalbumins were detected in high amounts in lower vertebrate white muscle [33], where they were believed to promote rapid relaxation from the active contractile state, a role that relies on parvalbumins' high affinity for calcium [34]. Subsequently, they were found, although in lesser amounts, in the fast-twitch skeletal muscles of higher vertebrates as well as in a variety of nonmuscle tissues, including testis, endocrine glands, skin, and neurons [35]. Parvalbumins possess 3EF-hand motifs: two that are able to chelate Ca^{2+} and Mg^{2+} and a third silent domain that forms a cap covering the hydrophobic surface of the two functional domains [36]. The parvalbumin family can be divided into two distinct phylogenetic lineages (alpha and beta). These two groups can be distinguished by their isoelectric points (pI,) (alpha: pI $\geq$5; beta: pI $\leq$4.5), sequence characteristics, affinities for Ca^{2+} and Mg^{2+}, cell-type–specific expression, and physiologic functions. Most muscles contain parvalbumin of only alpha or beta origin. Cod (Gad c 1) and salmon (Sal s 1) parvalbumin, for example, belong to the beta lineage and share significant similarity with parvalbumin of other fish species. Fish dark muscle is less allergenic than is white muscle because it contains much lower levels of parvalbumin. Thus, the dark muscle is implicated less in fish allergy than is the white muscle [37].

It is well known that parvalbumins are heat stable and resistant proteins because allergic patients react to cooked and raw fish. Furthermore, most patients showed stronger IgE binding to the calcium-bound form of parvalbumin [38,39].

Three-dimensional structure of calcium-binding allergens

The Protein Data Bank (http://www.rcsb.org/pdb/; release August 2006) contains only 3 entries for polcalcins: 1k9u (Phl p 7) [40], 1h4b (Bet v 4) [41], and 1pmz (Che a 3 [P. Verdino and colleagues, unpublished data, 2003]). In contrast, there are 35 entries for parvalbumins isolated from different animal species. The three-dimensional structure of parvalbumin has been determined from four fish species: pike (3pal) [42], silver hake (1bu3) [43], leopard shark (5pal) [44], and carp (4cpv) [45].

The three-dimensional structure of Phl p 7 was determined by x-ray crystallography at 0.175-Å resolution [40]. Phl p 7 occurs as a dimer assembly, which is in contrast to well-known EF-hand proteins (eg, calmodulin, parvalbumin, S-100 proteins). The dimer adopts a barrel-like structure with an extended hydrophobic cavity for ligand binding. The binding of calcium ions serves as a conformational switch between the open and closed dimeric forms of Phl p 7. The structural features of Phl p 7 suggest a role in pollen function; pollen tube germination and growth depend on calcium, and lipids are required for pollen tube guidance [46].

The structure of holo Bet v 4 was determined by heteronuclear nuclear magnetic resonance (NMR) spectroscopy [41], revealing a canonical 2EF-hand assembly in the open conformation. Unlike Phl p 7, the hydrodynamic parameters from NMR relaxation, NMR translational diffusion, and analytical ultracentrifugation indicated that apo and holo Bet v 4 predominantly are monomeric [41].

A structural comparison reveals some intrinsic features of the polcalcins. The monomeric Bet v 4 (1h4b) contains 2EF-hands, which are arranged symmetrically and bring the two calcium ions into spatial proximity (see Fig. 1). The monomer resembles the basic structural domain of the polcalcins. Two of these domains build up the dimeric Phl p 7 (1k9u), whereas four such domains are contained in the tetrameric Che a 3 (Fig. 2). In the oligomeric forms, a domain swapping of the polypeptide chains is observed; in Phl p 7 one half of chain A and one half of chain B builds up the basic structural domain (Fig. 3). The phenomenon of domain swapping was detected initially in diphtheria toxin [47], and is based on the fact that the interactions within the monomer are reused in the dimer. Structural superimposition clearly shows that the relative orientation of the EF-hands is the same in the monomeric and domain-swapped forms and that the spatial distance between the calcium ions differs only marginally.

Fish parvalbumins also consist of 2EF-hands. Fig. 4 shows the structural superimposition of carp parvalbumin (4cpv) and the monomeric polcalcin Bet v 4. Although the relative orientation of the EF-hands is similar, the remaining structure differs considerably (see Fig. 4), which might explain the lack of IgE cross-reactivity between plant and animal EF-hand calcium-binding allergens.

Influence of bound calcium on the three-dimensional structure and IgE-binding activity

Two conformation states of CBPs can be distinguished: a calcium-free form (apo-form) that represents the closed conformation, and a calcium-bound (holo-form) or open form of the molecule [1]. Calcium-binding allergens are divided into groups or subfamilies according to the number of conserved EF-hand motifs. The largest group contains 2EF-hand domains. Despite sequence similarity, some EF-hand motifs might be inactive with regards to their ability to bind calcium, as observed for one of the domains of the 3EF-hand allergen parvalbumin. Because it is known that the binding of calcium ions induces conformational changes in the structure (open and closed forms) and affects IgE binding to allergens, quantitative evaluation of the binding to calcium is of major importance to understand the allergenic/biologic activity of these proteins. Regarding IgE-binding activity, the calcium-depleted versions (apo-forms) of calcium-binding allergens are

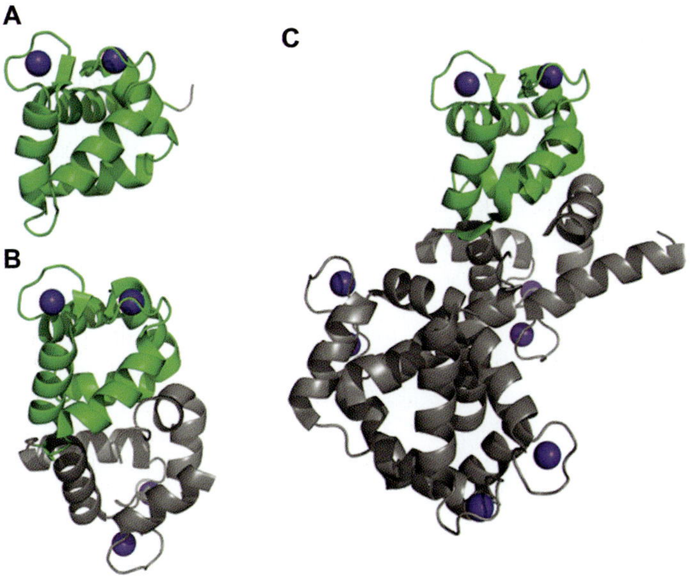

Fig. 2. Comparison of the three dimensional structure of Bet v 4 (*A*), Phl p 7 (*B*) and Che a 3 (*C*). Green indicates a single polcalcin domain. This figure was prepared with PyMOL (DeLano WL, The PyMOL Molecular Graphics System, 2002, http://www.pymol.org). Structure alignments were performed with SComPy (P. Lackner, PhD, unpublished in-house method, 2005).

less IgE reactive than are the calcium-bound (holo-) forms [1,38,48,49]. The switch between open and closed forms does not result in a major structural rearrangement, as observed for calmodulin upon peptide interaction; rather, it is restricted to local movements within the EF-hand motif. Besides IgE-binding activity, bound calcium also seems to affect heat stability [10,11,13].

To evaluate experimentally whether putative EF-hand motifs are able to bind calcium, $^{45}Ca^{2+}$ blot overlays or sodium doceyl sulfate-polyacrylamide gel electrophoresis band-shift assays can be performed. Conformational changes induced by binding or release of calcium ions can be analyzed by circular dichroism [10,11,13,18,50]. The calcium-binding activity of Bet v 4 was investigated by $^{45}Ca^{2+}$ blot overlays of wild-type and calcium-binding–deficient mutants [10]. In addition, the binding stoichiometry (number of moles of calcium bound per mole protein) and dissociation constant K_D of Bet v 4 was determined using circular dichroism [50]. In this way, it was possible to demonstrate that Bet v 4 is able to bind two calcium ions with high affinity, and, therefore, possesses two active EF-hands.

The three-dimensional structure of holo Bet v 4 revealed a canonical 2EF-hand assembly in the open conformation with interhelical angles closely resembling holo-calmodulin [41]. Further investigations of Bet v 4 indicated that both forms (apo and holo) predominantly are monomeric. This is in contrast to Phl p 7, whose apo- and holo-forms are exclusively

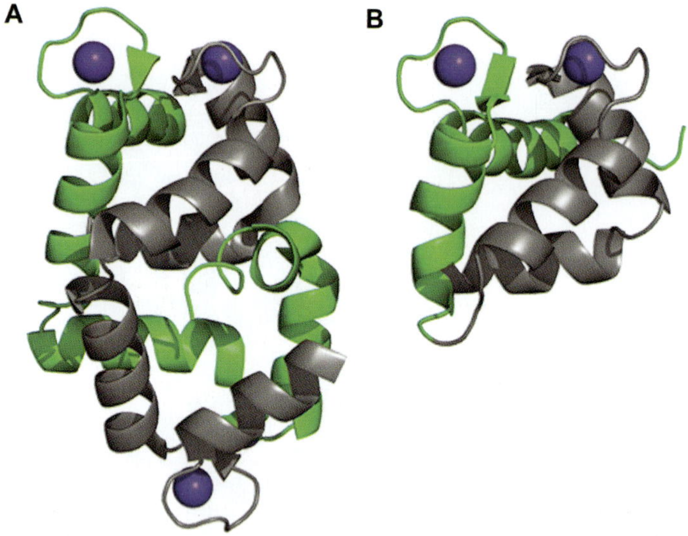

Fig. 3. Domain swapping in the dimeric polcalcin. Chain A of Phl p 7 is shown in green, chain B in gray (*left*). In the monomeric Bet v 4 (*right*), the structurally equivalent regions are shown in corresponding colors. This figure was prepared with PyMOL (DeLano WL, The PyMOL Molecular Graphics System, 2002, http://www.pymol.org). Structure alignments were performed with SComPy (P. Lackner, PhD, unpublished in-house method, 2005).

dimeric [40]. Because most IgE epitopes are unlikely to be affected by the domain-swapping dimerization, it might be assumed that canonical monomers and domain-swapped dimers may be of similar allergenicity; this explains the clinically observed IgE cross-reactivity between Bet v 4 and Phl p 7. Calcium-free form of Bet v 4 displayed reduced helicity and heat stability, as determined by circular dichroism. Also, a slightly increased hydrodynamic radius was observed, indicating a reversible structural transition upon calcium binding. These observations are in agreement with the reduced IgE-binding capacity of apo Bet v 4 [41].

Similarly to CBPs from pollen, depletion of calcium also drastically reduced IgE binding to fish parvalbumins. Calcium depletion of recombinant carp parvalbumin resulted in a strong reduction of the IgE-binding activity, which could be explained by calcium-induced changes in the protein conformation leading to exposure of amino acids that are buried in the apo-form of the allergen. Circular dichroism experiments showing differences between the apo- and the calcium-bound forms of carp Cyp c 1 were in agreement with this hypothesis [38].

IgE cross-reactivity

Cross-reactivity within the 2EF-hand family was demonstrated between timothy grass, Bermuda grass, ragweed, ash, and birch using rabbit anti–

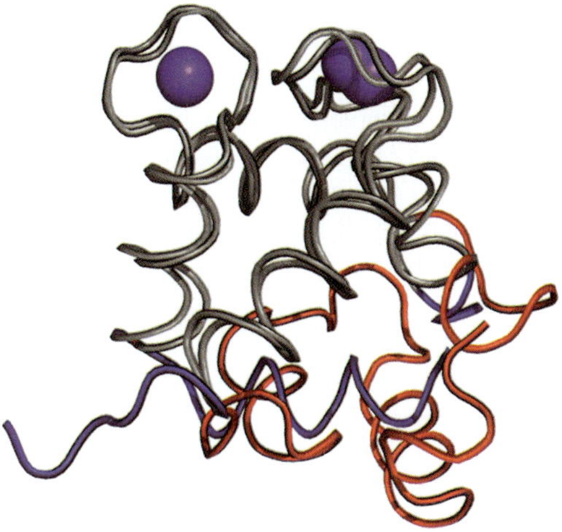

Fig. 4. Comparison of Carp parvalbumin and Bet v 4. The superimposed structures clearly show the high degree of similarity in the EF-hand regions (*gray*) and the dissimilarity in the remaining parts (*red and blue*). This figure was prepared with PyMOL (DeLano WL, The PyMOL Molecular Graphics System, 2002, http://www.pymol.org). Structure alignments were performed with SComPy (P. Lackner, PhD, unpublished in-house method, 2005).

rAln g 4 antiserum and IgE inhibition experiments [13,51]. The fact that patients who were sensitized to timothy grass pollen, olive, or mugwort pollen showed IgE reactivity to rBet v 4 or rAln g 4 suggested that they shared IgE epitopes with calcium-binding allergens in natural pollen extracts from various plants [10,11], and, therefore, were postulated to be cross-reactive allergens. Syr v 3, a 2EF-hand CBP from lilac, also reacted with Ole e 3–specific monoclonal antibodies and with IgE from patients who were allergic to olive-polcalcin; this demonstrated the presence of shared IgG and IgE epitopes [12]. Phl p 7 is one of the best-characterized polcalcins with respect to IgE cross-reactivity and three-dimensional structure [13,40,49]. Despite a low prevalence (10%) of IgE recognition, Phl p 7 showed high allergenic activity [13]. The calcium-bound form of the protein was recognized much more strongly by patients' IgE than was the calcium-depleted form [1]. Phl p 7 seems to contain most of the relevant IgE epitopes present in other calcium-binding allergen families [52]. It has been speculated that its allergenic activity might be related to its stable fold and the formation of dimers, which leads to a doubling of IgE epitopes and may give rise to potent cross-linking of effector cell-bound IgE antibodies [40]. In this respect, it would be interesting to compare the allergenic activities of monomeric Bet v 4, dimeric Phl p 7, and tetrameric Che a 3.

In a hierarchy of IgE cross-reactivity, rBet v 3 contained the least cross-reactive IgE epitopes compared with rPhl p7, rAln g 4, and rJun o 4 [52]. Amb a 10 from ragweed shows 55% sequence identity to Ole e 8, a 4EF-hand binding protein from olive pollen [18]. Amb a 10 also reacted with

Phl p 7–specific rabbit antiserum, demonstrating the presence of common IgG antibodies. ELISA data revealed that for some patients, depletion of calcium reduced IgE-binding activity. A subset of patients showed higher IgE reactivity after calcium depletion. Between 8% and 26% of tested patients showed IgE reactivity to Amb a 10, depending on the geographic area and the sensitization of the patients [7]. Testing preselected Phl p 7–positive polysensitized patients from Italy, the authors found that 70% of the patients cross-reacted with Amb a 10 (N. Wopfner, PhD, unpublished data, 2007).

To study whether the common EF-hand sequential motifs are involved in the IgE reactivity of Ole e 3 and Ole e 8, Ledesma and colleagues [48] performed indirect ELISA, ELISA inhibition, and immunoblotting experiments with sera from patients who were allergic to olive pollen. Different patterns for IgE and IgG recognition—as well as for dependency on bound calcium—was found for Ole e 3 and Ole e 8, respectively. The data suggested that, in general, EF-hand motifs are not highly cross-reactive allergenic epitopes.

Cod parvalbumin, Gad c 1 (formally allergen M) [31], is a major cross-reactive allergen among different fish species. Gad c 1 shares IgE-binding epitopes with various fish and even with frog parvalbumin. This cross-reactivity is of clinical relevance, because patients with a positive double-blind, placebo-controlled food challenge to cod also reacted to other fish species, such as herring, plaice, and mackerel [53,54]. Cod is among the most common offender, whereas salmon is tolerated best. Less than 50% of the patients who had cod allergy also reacted to salmon [55,56]. Another study on cross-reactivity of nine commonly consumed fish (cod, salmon, mackerel, tuna, herring, wolfish, halibut, pollack, and flounder) demonstrated that Gad c 1 and The c 1 (Alaska pollock) showed the highest IgE-binding affinities [55]. In this study, natural and recombinant parvalbumins from cod, salmon, and Alaska pollock were used in IgE- and IgG-inhibition experiments as well as for skin prick testing. The least allergenic fish were halibut, flounder, tuna, and mackerel [55]. IgE-binding patterns are more similar when fish species have closer phylogenetic relations and parvalbumins with higher amino acid sequence homology [57]. It should be noted that no added calcium was used in the ELISA-inhibition experiments or in the solutions for skin prick test [55,56]. It would be interesting to investigate the influence of bound calcium on the IgE recognition of parvalbumins in vivo.

Carp parvalbumin (Cyp c 1) is another well-characterized and cross-reactive fish allergen. Recombinant Cyp c 1 completely inhibited IgE binding to the natural protein and contained most of the IgE epitopes (almost 70%) present in allergen extracts of various fish species like tuna, cod, perch, and salmon [39].

To summarize, IgE recognition of calcium-binding allergens is influenced by binding or release of calcium ions, which induces conformational changes. Furthermore, different subfamilies of calcium-binding allergens have specific epitopes that could be involved in cross-reactivity among members of the same subfamily. Although there is cross-reactivity described within the subfamilies of calcium-binding allergens, there is no compelling evidence for IgE cross-reactivity between calcium-binding allergens from plants, fish, and humans [1]. Taken together, these findings suggest that the major IgE epitopes of calcium-binding allergens do not reside in the highly conserved calcium-binding regions, but are found in the less-conserved portions of the proteins [11,48,52]. Thus, despite extensive IgE cross-reactivity among CBPs belonging to the same subfamily, EF-hand calcium-binding sites of these allergens cannot be considered as general cross-reactive epitopes.

Summary

Because CBPs are ubiquitous inhalant allergens from plants, and fish parvalbumins are major food allergens, their complete characterization is of major importance. Allergens, such as Phl p 7 and Gad c 1or Cyp c 1, may be highly relevant for diagnosis and therapy. A comparison between allergens with 2EF-, 3EF-, and 4EF-hand domains showed that Phl p 7 is the most cross-reactive allergen among polcalcins [52]. Therefore, Phl p 7 could be used as a marker to identify multiple pollen-sensitized patients [52], whereas Gad c 1 or Cyp c 1 could be selected for diagnosis of fish allergy. Hom s 4 might be an interesting candidate to monitor chronic skin inflammation in atopic and nonatopic individuals [21]. Diagnostic tests containing these allergens/antigens could allow for the identification of most patients who are sensitized to calcium-binding allergens.

The knowledge concerning the influence of bound calcium on IgE reactivity could be used to engineer hypoallergenic CBPs for specific immunotherapy [49]. Mutations in the EF-hand motifs of these allergens to prevent binding of calcium ions would result in stable apo-forms with decreased IgE-binding activity.

Further studies using well-characterized recombinant calcium-binding allergens and other pan-allergens should be undertaken to better understand sensitization and IgE cross-reactivity and their clinical correlations.

References

[1] Valenta R, Hayek B, Seiberler S, et al. Calcium-binding allergens: from plants to man. Int Arch Allergy Immunol 1998;117(3):160–6.
[2] Grabarek Z. Structural basis for diversity of the EF-hand calcium-binding proteins. J Mol Biol 2006;359(3):509–25.
[3] Ikura M. Calcium binding and conformational response in EF-hand proteins. Trends Biochem Sci 1996;21(1):14–7.
[4] Kawasaki H, Kretsinger RH. Calcium-binding proteins. 1: EF-hands. Protein Profile 1994; 1(4):343–517.
[5] Aas K, Jebsen JW. Studies of hypersensitivity to fish. Partial purification and crystallization of a major allergenic component of cod. Int Arch Allergy Appl Immunol 1967;32(1):1–20.

[6] Coffee CJ, Bradshaw RA. Carp muscle calcium-binding protein. I. Characterization of the tryptic peptides and the complete amino acid sequence of component B. J Biol Chem 1973;248(9):3302–12.
[7] Asero R, Wopfner N, Gruber P, et al. *Artemisia* and *Ambrosia* hypersensitivity: co-sensitization or co-recognition? Clin Exp Allergy 2006;36(5):658–65.
[8] Barderas R, Villalba M, Pascual CY, et al. Profilin (Che a 2) and polcalcin (Che a 3) are relevant allergens of *Chenopodium album* pollen: isolation, amino acid sequences, and immunologic properties. J Allergy Clin Immunol 2004;113(6):1192–8.
[9] Batanero E, Villalba M, Ledesma A, et al. Ole e 3, an olive-tree allergen, belongs to a widespread family of pollen proteins. Eur J Biochem 1996;241(3):772–8.
[10] Engel E, Richter K, Obermeyer G, et al. Immunological and biological properties of Bet v 4, a novel birch pollen allergen with two EF-hand calcium-binding domains. J Biol Chem 1997; 272(45):28630–7.
[11] Hayek B, Vangelista L, Pastore A, et al. Molecular and immunologic characterization of a highly cross-reactive two EF-hand calcium-binding alder pollen allergen, Aln g 4: structural basis for calcium-modulated IgE recognition. J Immunol 1998;161(12):7031–9.
[12] Ledesma A, Barderas R, Westritschnig K, et al. A comparative analysis of the cross-reactivity in the polcalcin family including Syr v 3, a new member from lilac pollen. Allergy 2006; 61(4):477–84.
[13] Niederberger V, Hayek B, Vrtala S, et al. Calcium-dependent immunoglobulin E recognition of the apo- and calcium-bound form of a cross-reactive two EF-hand timothy grass pollen allergen, Phl p 7. FASEB J 1999;13(8):843–56.
[14] Smith PM, Xu H, Swoboda I, et al. Identification of a Ca2+ binding protein as a new Bermuda grass pollen allergen Cyn d 7: IgE cross-reactivity with oilseed rape pollen allergen Bra r 1. Int Arch Allergy Immunol 1997;114(3):265–71.
[15] Suphioglu C, Ferreira F, Knox RB. Molecular cloning and immunological characterisation of Cyn d 7, a novel calcium-binding allergen from Bermuda grass pollen. FEBS Lett 1997; 402(2-3):167–72.
[16] Toriyama K, Okada T, Watanabe M, et al. A cDNA clone encoding an IgE-binding protein from *Brassica* anther has significant sequence similarity to Ca(2+)-binding proteins. Plant Mol Biol 1995;29(6):1157–65.
[17] Seiberler S, Scheiner O, Kraft D, et al. Characterization of a birch pollen allergen, Bet v III, representing a novel class of Ca2+ binding proteins: specific expression in mature pollen and dependence of patients' IgE binding on protein-bound Ca2+. EMBO J 1994; 13(15):3481–6.
[18] Ledesma A, Villalba M, Rodriguez R. Cloning, expression and characterization of a novel four EF-hand Ca(2+)-binding protein from olive pollen with allergenic activity. FEBS Lett 2000;466(1):192–6.
[19] Tinghino R, Barletta B, Palumbo S, et al. Molecular characterization of a cross-reactive *Juniperus oxycedrus* pollen allergen, Jun o 2: a novel calcium-binding allergen. J Allergy Clin Immunol 1998;101(6):772–7.
[20] Bugajska-Schretter A, Elfman L, Fuchs T, et al. Parvalbumin, a cross-reactive fish allergen, contains IgE-binding epitopes sensitive to periodate treatment and Ca2+ depletion. J Allergy Clin Immunol 1998;101(1):67–74.
[21] Aichberger KJ, Mittermann I, Reininger R, et al. Hom s 4, an IgE-reactive autoantigen belonging to a new subfamily of calcium-binding proteins, can induce Th cell type 1-mediated autoreactivity. J Immunol 2005;175(2):1286–94.
[22] Rathore KS, Cork RJ, Robinson KR. A cytoplasmic gradient of Ca2+ is correlated with the growth of lily pollen tubes. Dev Biol 1991;148(2):612–9.
[23] Berchtold MW, Brinkmeier H, Muntener M. Calcium ion in skeletal muscle: its crucial role for muscle function, plasticity, and disease. Physiol Rev 2000;80(3):1215–65.
[24] Radauer C, Breiteneder H. Pollen allergens are restricted to few protein families and show distinct patterns of species distribution. J Allergy Clin Immunol 2006;117(1):141–7.

[25] Wopfner N, Gadermaier G, Egger M, et al. The spectrum of allergens in ragweed and mugwort pollen. Int Arch Allergy Immunol 2005;138(4):337–46.
[26] Stumvoll S, Westritschnig K, Lidholm J, et al. Identification of cross-reactive and genuine *Parietaria judaica* pollen allergens. J Allergy Clin Immunol 2003;111(5):974–9.
[27] Quiralte J, Florido F, Arias de Saavedra JM, et al. Olive allergen-specific IgE responses in patients with *Olea europaea* pollinosis. Allergy 2002;57(Suppl 71):47–52.
[28] Moverare R, Westritschnig K, Svensson M, et al. Different IgE reactivity profiles in birch pollen-sensitive patients from six European populations revealed by recombinant allergens: an imprint of local sensitization. Int Arch Allergy Immunol 2002;128(4):325–35.
[29] Ledesma A, Villalba M, Vivanco F, et al. Olive pollen allergen Ole e 8: identification in mature pollen and presence of Ole e 8-like proteins in different pollens. Allergy 2002; 57(1):40–3.
[30] Aas K. Societal implications of food allergy: coping with atopic disease in children and adolescents. Ann Allergy 1987;59(5):194–9.
[31] Aas K, Elsayed SM. Characterization of a major allergen (cod). Effect of enzymic hydrolysis on the allergenic activity. J Allergy 1969;44(6):333–43.
[32] Elsayed S, Aas K. Characterization of a major allergen (cod). Observations on effect of denaturation on the allergenic activity. J Allergy 1971;47(5):283–91.
[33] Pechere JF. The significance of parvalbumins among muscular calcium proteins. Amsterdam: Elsevier; 1997.
[34] Gillis JM, Thomason D, Lefevre J, et al. Parvalbumins and muscle relaxation: a computer simulation study. J Muscle Res Cell Motil 1982;3(4):377–98.
[35] Lehky P, Blum HE, Stein EA, et al. Isolation and characterization of parvalbumins from the skeletal muscle of higher vertebrates. J Biol Chem 1974;249(13):4332–4.
[36] Kretsinger RH, Nockolds CE. Carp muscle calcium-binding protein. II. Structure determination and general description. J Biol Chem 1973;248(9):3313–26.
[37] Kobayashi A, Tanaka H, Hamada Y, et al. Comparison of allergenicity and allergens between fish white and dark muscles. Allergy 2006;61(3):357–63.
[38] Bugajska-Schretter A, Grote M, Vangelista L, et al. Purification, biochemical, and immunological characterisation of a major food allergen: different immunoglobulin E recognition of the apo- and calcium-bound forms of carp parvalbumin. Gut 2000;46(5):661–9.
[39] Swoboda I, Bugajska-Schretter A, Verdino P, et al. Recombinant carp parvalbumin, the major cross-reactive fish allergen: a tool for diagnosis and therapy of fish allergy. J Immunol 2002;168(9):4576–84.
[40] Verdino P, Westritschnig K, Valenta R, et al. The cross-reactive calcium-binding pollen allergen, Phl p 7, reveals a novel dimer assembly. EMBO J 2002;21(19):5007–16.
[41] Neudecker P, Nerkamp J, Eisenmann A, et al. Solution structure, dynamics, and hydrodynamics of the calcium-bound cross-reactive birch pollen allergen Bet v 4 reveal a canonical monomeric two EF-hand assembly with a regulatory function. J Mol Biol 2004;336(5):1141–57.
[42] Declercq JP, Tinant B, Parello J, et al. Ionic interactions with parvalbumins. Crystal structure determination of pike 4.10 parvalbumin in four different ionic environments. J Mol Biol 1991;220(4):1017–39.
[43] Richardson RC, King NM, Harrington DJ, et al. X-Ray crystal structure and molecular dynamics simulations of silver hake parvalbumin (Isoform B). Protein Sci 2000;9(1): 73–82.
[44] Roquet F, Declercq JP, Tinant B, et al. Crystal structure of the unique parvalbumin component from muscle of the leopard shark (*Triakis semifasciata*). The first X-ray study of an alpha-parvalbumin. J Mol Biol 1992;223(3):705–20.
[45] Kumar VD, Lee L, Edwards BF. Refined crystal structure of calcium-liganded carp parvalbumin 4.25 at 1.5-A resolution. Biochemistry 1990;29(6):1404–12.
[46] Franklin-Tong VE. Signaling in pollination. Curr Opin Plant Biol 1999;2(6):490–5.
[47] Bennett MJ, Choe S, Eisenberg D. Domain swapping: entangling alliances between proteins. Proc Natl Acad Sci U S A 1994;91(8):3127–31.

[48] Ledesma A, Gonzalez E, Pascual CY, et al. Are Ca2+-binding motifs involved in the immunoglobin E-binding of allergens? Olive pollen allergens as model of study. Clin Exp Allergy 2002;32(10):1476–83.

[49] Westritschnig K, Focke M, Verdino P, et al. Generation of an allergy vaccine by disruption of the three-dimensional structure of the cross-reactive calcium-binding allergen, Phl p 7. J Immunol 2004;172(9):5684–92.

[50] Hebenstreit D, Ferreira F. Structural changes in calcium-binding allergens: use of circular dichroism to study binding characteristics. Allergy 2005;60(9):1208–11.

[51] Niederberger V, Purohit A, Oster JP, et al. The allergen profile of ash (*Fraxinus excelsior*) pollen: cross-reactivity with allergens from various plant species. Clin Exp Allergy 2002; 32(6):933–41.

[52] Tinghino R, Twardosz A, Barletta B, et al. Molecular, structural, and immunologic relationships between different families of recombinant calcium-binding pollen allergens. J Allergy Clin Immunol 2002;109(2):314–20.

[53] Bernhisel-Broadbent J, Scanlon SM, Sampson HA. Fish hypersensitivity. I. In vitro and oral challenge results in fish-allergic patients. J Allergy Clin Immunol 1992;89(3):730–7.

[54] Pascual C, Martin Esteban M, Crespo JF. Fish allergy: evaluation of the importance of cross-reactivity. J Pediatr 1992;121(5):S29–34.

[55] Van Do T, Elsayed S, Florvaag E, et al. Allergy to fish parvalbumins: studies on the cross-reactivity of allergens from 9 commonly consumed fish. J Allergy Clin Immunol 2005;116(6): 1314–20.

[56] Van Do T, Hordvik I, Endresen C, et al. Expression and analysis of recombinant salmon parvalbumin, the major allergen in Atlantic salmon (*Salmo salar*). Scand J Immunol 1999;50(6): 619–25.

[57] Elsayed S, Apold J. Immunochemical analysis of cod fish allergen M: locations of the immunoglobulin binding sites as demonstrated by the native and synthetic peptides. Allergy 1983; 38(7):449–59.

ELSEVIER
SAUNDERS

Immunol Allergy Clin N Am
27 (2007) 45–63

IMMUNOLOGY
AND ALLERGY
CLINICS
OF NORTH AMERICA

Pollen NAD(P)H Oxidases and Their Contribution to Allergic Inflammation

Nilesh G. Dharajiya, MD[a], Attila Bacsi, PhD[b], Istvan Boldogh, DMB, PhD[c], Sanjiv Sur, MD[d,*]

[a]*NHLBI Proteomics Center, Department of Biochemistry and Molecular Biology, University of Texas Medical Branch, 301 University Boulevard, Galveston, TX 77555-1083, USA*

[b]*Institute of Immunology, University of Debrecen, 98. Nagyerdei Boulevard, Debrecen, Hungary H-4021*

[c]*Department of Microbiology and Immunology, University of Texas Medical Branch, 301 University Boulevard, Galveston, TX 77555-1083, USA*

[d]*NHLBI Proteomics Center, Divisions of Allergy Pulmonary Immunology Critical Care and Sleep, Department of Internal Medicine, University of Texas Medical Branch, 301 University Boulevard, Galveston, TX 77555-1083, USA*

The Latin definition of pollen is *fine powder*. Analogous to sperms of the animal kingdom, pollens are plant male germ cells containing haploid chromosomes. Released from the anther of the flower, pollens reach the plant female reproductive organ (stigma) by means of wind, water, or insects in a process termed *pollination*. Pollens not only carry genetic information from anther to stigma but also have a broad impact on human health. Inhaling pollens can induce symptoms of seasonal asthma and allergic rhinitis in sensitized individuals [1,2]. Because of their microscopic size, some pollen grains and subpollen particles can penetrate lower airways and induce allergic airway inflammation [3,4]. Pollens contain a large number of antigenic proteins, such as the pectate lyase Amb a 1 in ragweed; defensin-like Art v 1 in mugwort; Pla l 1 in plantain; Che a 1 in goosefoot; and nonspecific lipid transfer proteins Par j 1 and Par j 2 in pellitory [5]. These antigenic proteins are processed in antigen-presenting cells and presented to T-helper

This work was supported by grants from the National Institutes of Health (#1R01 HL071163, SS), the NIAID Program Project Grant (#1P01 AI062885, SS & IB), and the National Heart, Lung, and Blood Institute Proteomics Initiative (#N01-HV28184, SS). The authors do not have any conflicts of interest in terms of relationships with commercial companies.

* Corresponding author.
E-mail address: sasur@utmb.edu (S. Sur).

0889-8561/07/$ - see front matter
doi:10.1016/j.iac.2006.11.007

cells, thereby triggering an adaptive immune response culminating in allergic inflammation.

In addition to these antigens, pollens contain myriad other proteins, some with enzymatic activities. The plasma membrane of plant cells contains NADPH oxidases that are similar to the inducible NADPH oxidase complex in the plasma membrane of mammalian phagocytes [6–9]. These plant oxidases play a critical role in vital physiologic functions, including defense against pathogens [10–12], growth and development [8,13,14], and expansion of cells in the root hairs [15]. The authors discovered the presence of NADPH oxidase activity in pollen grains of various plants, including grasses, weeds, and trees [16]. This article provides an overview of mammalian and plant NADPH oxidase and generation of reactive oxygen species. The role of NADPH oxidase–induced oxidative stress in allergic inflammation is also described.

Historical perspectives

Oxygen (O_2) constitutes 21% of the atmospheric air. O_2 is an essential element of survival for all animals and plants except anaerobic organisms. Aerobic energy production uses an O_2-dependent electron transport chain present in eukaryotic mitochondria. The advantage of the aerobic respiration can be ascertained from the fact that aerobic glycolysis produces 36 ATP molecules compared with only 2 ATP molecules produced by anaerobic glycolysis. However, this enormous energy source has a caveat: O_2 is a toxic and mutagenic. Aerobic organisms survive in the presence of O_2 only because they have developed mechanisms that eliminate toxic O_2 products and repair damaged biomolecules such as DNA.

Phagocytic host defense is a component of the innate immune system and a first line of defense against invading microorganisms. Phagocytes generate reactive oxygen species (ROS) that kill the microorganisms. However, this response is nonspecific and bystander host cells are also damaged, analogous to collateral damage in military terms. In 1883, Metchnikoff [17] performed pioneering work in the field of phagocytic host defense by showing that when transparent starfish larvae were pierced with a thorn, cells surrounded the sharp thorn. Fifty years later, Baldridge and Gerard [18] showed that when neutrophils were exposed to bacteria, a transient but sharp increase in O_2 uptake by the cells occurred. They termed this phenomenon *respiratory burst*, because they attributed the increase to oxidative phosphorylation by the mitochondria. However, in 1959, Sbarra and Karnovsky [19] reported that mitochondrial poison cyanide had no effect on respiratory burst, ruling out the long-held notion that mitochondria were responsible for increased oxygen demand when the neutrophils were engaged in killing bacteria. These reports, in addition to the discovery that common human bacterial pathogens are not killed in an anaerobic environment despite their normal phagocytosis [20], fueled the search for a molecular component in the cell that was responsible for oxygen uptake and host defense against bacteria. Later researchers discovered that activated neutrophils generated hydrogen peroxide (H_2O_2) and hypochlorous acid (HOCl). Myeloperoxidase enzyme present in neutrophils catalyzed the reaction between H_2O_2 and chloride ions to generate HOCl [21], commercially available as Clorox (The Clorox Company, Oakland, California).

The last piece in the puzzle was solved with the observation of an inherited syndrome in which patients were predisposed to frequent infections by an otherwise nonpathogenic bacterium, such as *Serratia marcescens*. This syndrome was initially believed to be a neoplastic condition because of formation of multiple granulomas infiltrated by macrophages and lymphocytes in these patients. This disease was termed *chronic granulomatous disease* (CGD) because of its pathologic manifestation of granulomas in multiple organs. Further studies showed that neutrophils from patients who had CGD were incapable of killing bacteria and could not generate H_2O_2 [22]. Around the same time, investigators discovered that biologic systems could convert O_2 into superoxide anions ($O_2^{\cdot-}$) [23–25], and Babior and colleagues [26] showed that $O_2^{\cdot-}$ is responsible for bacterial killing, indicating the role of $O_2^{\cdot-}$ in the pathogenesis of CGD. Different subunits of NADPH oxidase were characterized and molecular defects of these subunits were identified in patients who had CGD. Most patients who have CGD inherit the disease in an X-linked recessive manner with defects in the membrane-bound NADPH oxidase subunit, gp91^{phox} (phox for *phagocytic oxidase*). Mutations in other NADPH oxidase subunits, such as p47, p67, and p22, were identified in an autosomal-recessive form of CGD.

Mammalian NADPH oxidase

NADPH oxidase is an enzyme present in phagocytic cells such as macrophages, neutrophils, and eosinophils [27–29]. Eukaryotic NADPH oxidase is a complex multimolecular enzyme that transports electrons across the plasma membrane to convert O_2 into $O_2^{\cdot-}$. NADPH oxidase is composed of cytosolic and membrane subunits (Fig. 1). The cytosolic components are p47^{phox}, p40^{phox}, p67^{phox}, and the small G-proteins Rac2 and Cdc42 [30–32]. The membrane-bound components gp91^{phox} and p22^{phox} form a heterodimeric structure known as cytochrome b_{558} (cyt b558) [33]. On cell stimulation, the p47^{phox}, p40^{phox}, and p67^{phox} translocate and form a complex with membrane-bound cyt b558 in 1:1:1:1 stoichiometry [34]. Small GTPase proteins, such as Rac2 and Cdc42, also participate in activating the enzyme complex [35]. Fig. 1 provides a conceptual model of NADPH oxidase components and its activation-induced assembly in the membrane. A brief overview of each NADPH oxidase component is presented here.

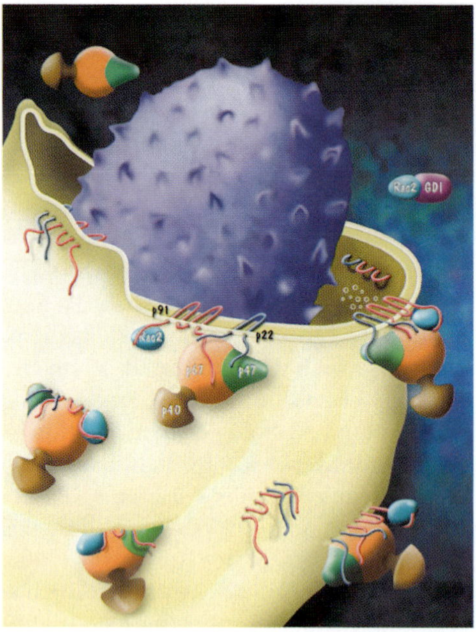

Fig. 1. Schematic illustration of NADPH oxidase in action. NADPH oxidase components are shown in the context of intact phagosome. Cytosolic and membrane subunits are in various stages of assembly to form activated NADPH oxidase on the membrane in response to bacterial stimulus. gp91^{phox} and p22^{phox} are shown as pink and blue helices anchored to the membrane. Rac2, GDP dissociation inhibitor (GDI), p40^{phox}, p47^{phox}, and p67^{phox} are coded by color and shape. Ingested bacterium is shown in purple. (*Reproduced from* Bokoch GM, Knaus UG. NADPH oxidase: not just for leukocytes anymore! Trends Biochem Sci 2003;28(9):502–8; with permission.)

Cytosolic subunits of NADPH oxidase

p47^{phox}

p47^{phox} is 390-amino-acid peptide containing phox homology (PX), SH3, autoinhibitory, and proline-rich region domains (Fig. 2). The PX domain is named after its presence in p47^{phox} and p40^{phox} [36]. This domain is present in the *N*-terminus of p47^{phox} and facilitates its anchoring to phosphatidylinositol-3,4 bisphosphate [PI(3)P2] and adjacent phosphatidylinositol-3 phosphate present in the cell membrane [37]. A tandem repeat of two SH3 domains occurs, the first of which binds to a proline-rich sequence in the *C*-terminus of p22^{phox}, and the second binds to a proline-rich region of p67^{phox} (see Fig. 2; Fig. 3). An autoinhibitory domain present in the *C*-terminal region of p47^{phox} exhibits intramolecular interaction with the SH3 domain, preventing it from interacting with p22^{phox} of cyt b558 (see Fig. 3) [38]. This masking effect ensures the inadvertent activation of NADPH oxidase and production of oxygen radicals.

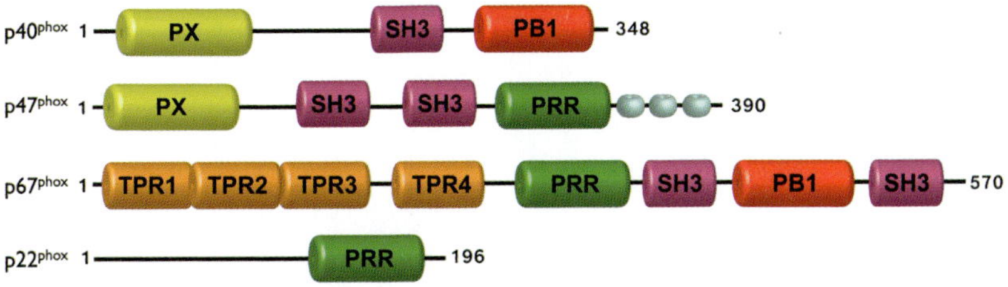

Fig. 2. Structural domains of NADPH oxidase subunits. The domain structures of p40^{phox}, p47^{phox}, p67^{phox}, and p22^{phox} are shown in illustrative cartoon. Different domains in phox subunits are color coded. Phosphorylation sites in p47^{phox} are shown as light blue spheres. The length of each subunit is approximated to total amino acids present in the proteins. PB1, phagocytic oxidase and Bem 1; PRR, proline-rich region; PX, Phox homolog; SH3, Src homology 3 domain; TPR, tetratricopepide repeat.

Activation of the cell leads to phosphorylation of serines in the autoinhibitory domain, thereby disrupting its association with the SH3 domain and making it accessible for interaction with p22^{phox} (Fig. 4) [38]. The proline-rich region of the p47^{phox} domain binds to the SH3 domain in the

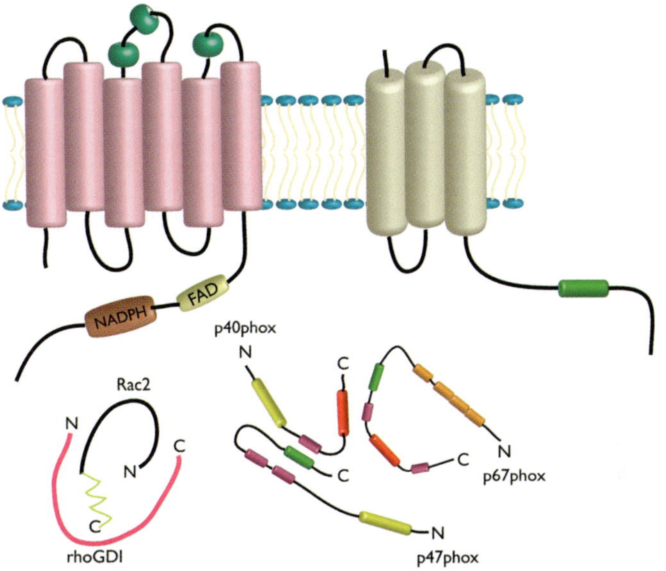

Fig. 3. NADPH oxidase components in resting state. Cytoplasmic and membrane bound subunits are shown in resting state. The pink- and cream-colored barrels indicate predicted transmembrane helices of gp91^{phox} and p22^{phox}, respectively. Glycosylation sites in gp91^{phox} are shown as green spheres. The FAD and NADPH binding sites in gp91^{phox} are shown as light yellow and brown tubules. Rac2 bound to RhoGDI (guanine nucleotide dissociation inhibitor) is shown as black and pink think lines. The thin green line on the *C*-terminus of Rac2 represents geranyl–geranyl moiety, which facilitates its association with membrane. P40^{phox}, p47^{phox}, and p67^{phox} are displayed according to the structural model shown in Fig. 2. Interaction between p40^{phox} and p47^{phox} through the SH3 and PRR domains are shown.

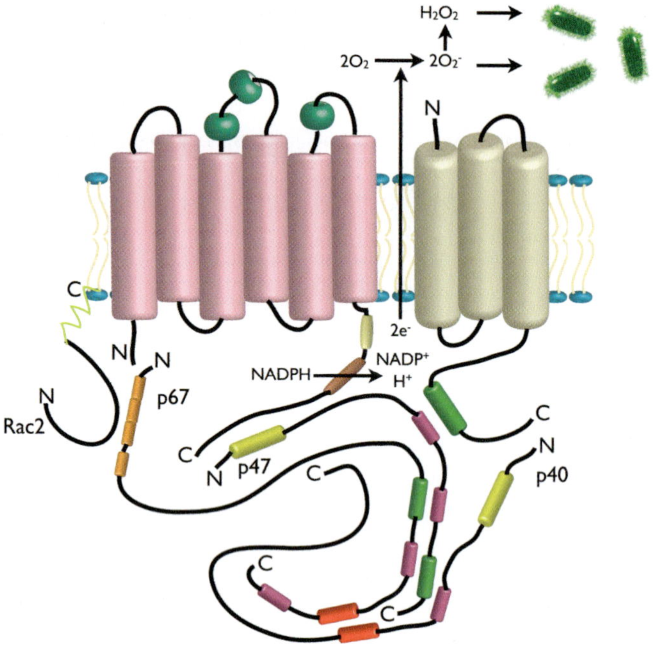

Fig. 4. Activation-induced NADPH oxidase subunit assembly in membrane. In the active state, RhoGDI dissociates from Rac2, and the latter then anchors to the membrane. P47^{phox} associates with the *C*-terminal end of gp91^{phox} and with p22^{phox} through its SH3 domain. p67^{phox} interacts with Rac2 through its TPR domains on the *N*-terminus, and with p47^{phox} through SH3 and PRR domain interactions. p40^{phox} weakly associates with p47^{phox} through SH3 and PRR interaction and with p67^{phox} through PB1 interaction. This assembly leads to activation of the NADPH oxidase complex, which converts NADPH to NADP+, and resulting electrons are transported across the membrane, converting molecular oxygen to superoxide. Superoxides are eventually converted to H_2O_2 by superoxide dismutase and together these ROS mediate the killing of pathogens.

C-terminus of p67^{phox} in a tail-to-tail interaction (Fig. 4). Phosphorylation of p47^{phox} is a prerequisite for its membrane translocation and interaction with p22^{phox}. Mutations in p47^{phox}, including the PX domain, have been associated with CGD [39,40]. However, in a cell-free system, the presence of p47^{phox} is not required when p67^{phox} and Rac2 are in excess [41]. Therefore, p47^{phox} mainly functions as an adaptor protein that binds to p67 and p40 and translocates them to the cell membrane.

p67^{phox}

p67^{phox} is a 526-amino-acid protein with tetratricopeptide repeat (TPR), activation, proline-rich region, SH3, and PB1 domains (see Fig. 2). Four TPR domains in the *N*-terminal of p67^{phox} interact with Rac in a guanosine triphosphate (GTP)–dependent manner (see Fig. 4) [42]. Once phosphorylated, the activation domain binds to gp91^{phox} and regulates electron flow from NADPH to cyt b558 [43]. The presence of amino acids 199–210 is an absolute requirement for $O_2^{\cdot-}$ production in a cell-free system [44]. The proline-rich region domain of $p67^{phox}$ binds to a second SH3 domain of $p47^{phox}$. Two SH3 domains are found in $p67^{phox}$, one of which binds to the proline-rich region of $p47^{phox}$. The PB1 domain is named after its presence in phagocytic oxidase and Bem 1 proteins [45]. PB1 is essentially a protein–protein interaction motif that associates with PB1 in $p40^{phox}$ to form a heterodimer (see Fig. 4). Translocation of $p67^{phox}$, $p40^{phox}$, and Rac2 from cytosol to membrane-bound cyt b558 involves $p67^{phox}$ phosphorylation (see Figs. 3 and 4). $p67^{phox}$ mutations are rare in CGD and, when present, result in decreased oxidase production [46].

p40^phox

$p40^{phox}$ is a 339-amino-acid protein and the last subunit of the NADPH oxidase to be identified by copurification with $p47^{phox}$ and $p67^{phox}$. It is composed of PX, SH3, and PB1 domains (see Fig. 2). The PX domain binds to PI(3)P2 and facilitates oxidase assembly in cell membrane. The SH3 domain of $p40^{phox}$ interacts weakly with proline-rich region in $p47^{phox}$ [47]. $p40^{phox}$ contains a PB1 domain similar to $p67^{phox}$ that mediates interaction between these proteins (see Fig. 4). The overall role of $p40^{phox}$ remains under debate, although it has been reported to both up-regulate and down-regulate activity of NADPH oxidase [48,49]. At least in the cell-free system, $p40^{phox}$ is not required for oxidase activity [50].

G-proteins

Rac and Cdc42 are G-proteins that belong to the Rho subfamily of proteins, which regulates a wide spectrum of functions such as intracellular signaling, cytoskeletal organization, generation of ROS, and cell growth. Three isoforms of Rac have been identified, with Rac1 ubiquitously expressed and Rac2 largely restricted to hemopoietic cells [51]. The predominant isoform in human neutrophils is Rac2. The association between NADPH oxidase and G-proteins was initially suspected because guanine nucleotides could stimulate NADPH oxidase [52]. In a resting state, Rac2 is bound to guanine-nucleotide dissociation inhibitor (GDI), inhibiting its interaction with the NADPH oxidase subunits p67 and cyt b558 (see Fig. 3). Appropriate stimuli induce dissociation of Rac2 from GDI and promote exchange of guanosine diphosphate (GDP) for GTP with the help of guanine-nucleotide exchange factors (GEF) [53]. Structural studies have shown the presence of switch I and II regions and an insert domain on Rac2. Interaction between Rac2 and cyt b558 is mediated through an insert region and is GTP-dependent. In the GTP-bound state, Rac2, through its switch I or effector region, can associate with the TPR domain of $p67^{phox}$ (see Fig. 4).

The association of Rac2 and cytosolic subunits of NADPH oxidase with cyt b558 creates machinery for electron transfer from NADPH to O_2 involving two steps. In the first step, electrons are transferred from NADPH to the flavin adenine dinucleotide (FAD) moiety of cytochrome, and in the second phase, electrons are passed from FAD to heme in cyt b558 and then to molecular oxygen to form $O_2^{\cdot -}$ [54]. A mutation in human Rac2 was identified that inhibits its association with GTP, resulting in decreased chemotaxis, $O_2^{\cdot -}$ production, and azurophilic secretion [55].

Membrane-associated NADPH oxidase subunits

Cytochrome b_{558}

Cyt b558 is a flavohemoprotein composed of two subunits, gp91^{phox} and p22^{phox}. Cyt b558 is named because of its absorption peak at 558 nm. It is also known as Cyt b-245 because of its midpoint potential of −245 mV. Although the molecular weight of the large subunit gp91^{phox} is actually 65 kd, the extensive glycosylation process creates a diffuse band of approximately 91 kd on sodium dodecylsulfate (SDS) gels. Hydrophobic domains in the *N*-terminal region of gp91^{phox} form the membrane-spanning domains, whereas the hydrophilic *C*-terminal domain interacts with the p47^{phox} and heme moieties (see Figs. 3 and 4). Flavohemoprotein derives its name from the presence of FAD, which receives electrons from NADPH and two heme prosthetic groups that mediate further electron transfer to O_2. The presence of FAD is mandatory for $O_2^{\cdot -}$ generation, because removing FAD results in the loss of oxidase activity, and returning it restores the activity. Thus, gp91^{phox} contains all the components required for electron transfer, a concept supported by the report that gp91^{phox} functions similar to the H^+ channel and permits electron transport across the cell membrane [56]. Mutations of gp91^{phox} are associated with an X-linked CGD [57]. A phenotype similar to CGD is observed in gp91^{phox} knockout mice [58].

The p22^{phox} is a 21-kd protein that associates with gp91^{phox} in 1:1 stoichiometry (see Fig. 2). The heterodimer formation enhances the maturation and structural stability of gp91^{phox} [59]. The presence of three transmembrane α-helices in the *N*-terminal region of p22^{phox} forms the membrane insertion region, whereas the cytosolic *C*-terminal contains a proline-rich region that can interact with the SH3 domain of p47^{phox} (see Figs. 3 and 4). Mutations in p22^{phox} are associated with autosomal-recessive CGD [60].

Plant NAD(P)H oxidase

Plants are confined to a physical location because of their sessile growth and life. Therefore, developing defense mechanisms against broad range of biotic and abiotic stresses is critical. Pathogenic bacteria, viruses, and fungi are among the most dangerous threats to plant survival. Coevolution of plants with various pathogens has enabled them to develop many different defense strategies through continuous exchange of molecular information between the groups. Some of the common defense reactions are cell-wall reinforcement and the production of antimicrobial agents, hydrolytic enzymes, and phytoalexins. The presence of an external threat is perceived through recognition of signal molecules known as *elicitors* released by microorganisms or plant cells in response to pathogens. Whether plants acquire resistance and clear the pathogen or become susceptible to the pathogen and develop disease depends largely on the speed and extent of intracellular signaling and the accumulation of defense products.

The defense responses are mainly regulated at transcription level by defense-related genes, resulting in delayed response time. However, occasionally the defense reactions primarily involve activation of preexisting components rather than de novo synthesis using the biosynthetic machinery of the cell. One of the most striking examples of this immediate response is the rapid, transient, and large release of ROS, termed *oxidative burst*, which is analogous to respiratory burst in mammalian cells. The function of ROS is not just limited to defense response; subsequent studies identified its vital role in a broad range of physiologic processes in plants, such as removal of aleurone layer, stomatal closure, allelopathy, root elongation, and gravitropism [15,61–64]. Current understanding of the mechanisms of respiratory burst largely derived from studies of effects of elicitors on suspension-culture plant cells. Doke [65] showed for the first time that potato tuber discs exposed to an avirulent strain of *Phytopthera infestans* generated an NAD(P)H-dependent rapid burst of ROS production. Furthermore, using a cytochrome C assay and nitroblue tetrazolium reduction assay, these investigators identified $O_2^{\cdot -}$ as the major ROS released from the cells. Infection with a virulent strain of the same pathogen failed to induce ROS. Later, Jabs and colleagues [66] identified that diphenylene iodonium (DPI), an inhibitor of mammalian NAD(P)H oxidase, abrogated this ROS generation. Cell fractionation studies indicated the presence of NADPH-dependent ROS-inducing activities in plasma-membrane, similar to the presence of cell-membrane components of human NAD(P)H oxidase [67]. Collectively, these studies provided presumptive evidence that NAD(P)H oxidase exists in plants.

Respiratory burst oxidase homologues

Groom and colleagues [68] identified the first plant NAD(P)H oxidase gene in *Oryza sativa* and termed it *respiratory burst oxidase homologue* (*Rboh*) because of its homology to human *gp91^{phox}*. Several *Rboh* genes were later identified in many other plant species, including *Arabidopsis*, tomato, tobacco, and potato [11,69–71]. *A. thaliana Rboh* (*Atrboh*) genes are very well characterized and are described here as representative of similar *Rboh* genes in other plant species. Currently, 10 *Atrboh* genes have been identified that code for highly similar proteins [69]. All Rboh proteins contain six transmembrane domains followed by FAD and NAD(P)H domains near their *C*-terminal end. The *N*-terminal regions boast two EF hands with a structural similarity to mammalian NOX5 and DUOX1 proteins. The EF hands can bind Ca^{2+}, allowing direct regulation of oxidase activity and $O_2^{\cdot-}$ production through Ca^{2+} signaling [12]. This mechanism contrasts with that for mammalian gp91^{phox}, which lacks the EF hands and therefore depends on association with cytoplasmic components of NAD(P)H oxidase to generate $O_2^{\cdot-}$. Unlike mammalian gp91^{phox}, the Rboh crystal structure is not solved; however, a hypothetical model of its organization in plant cell membrane is shown in Fig. 5. Another common feature between mammalian and plant NAD(P)H oxidase exists in the form of regulatory proteins. Several Rho-like proteins (ROPs, also known as RAC) have been identified in different species of plants that differentially regulate activity of NAD(P)H oxidase during defense signaling and other physiologic processes [72–74].

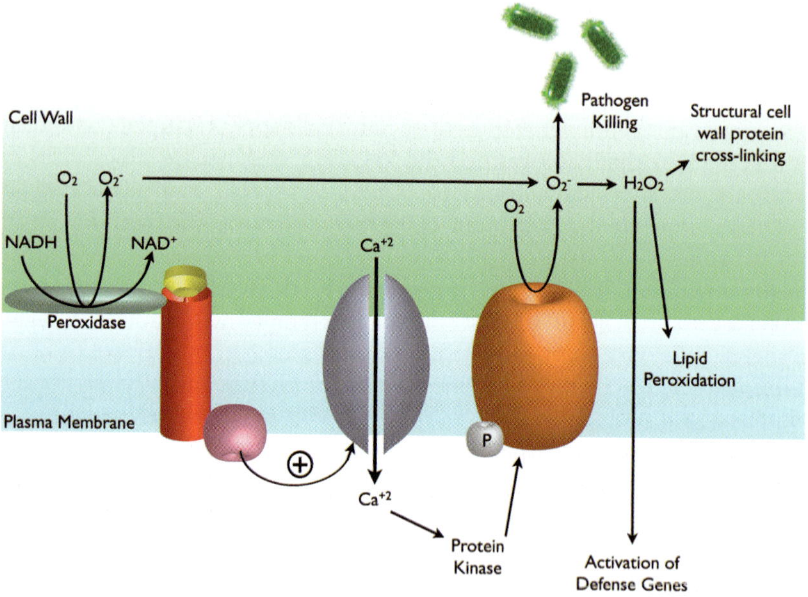

Fig. 5. A speculative model of plant NAD(P)H oxidase. Binding of elicitor (*yellow*) to its receptor (*red barrel*) in the membrane may stimulate membrane-associated peroxidases (*green disk*) through unknown mechanisms, which result in $O_2^{\cdot-}$ synthesis. Alternatively, elicitor receptors coupled to G-proteins (*pink sphere*), and increased intracellular Ca^{2+} caused by Ca^{2+} channel opening (*gray channel*) and activation of protein kinase, may activate membrane-bound NAD(P)H oxidase (*orange*) through phosphorylation (*gray sphere with P*), resulting in conversion of O_2 to $O_2^{\cdot-}$. The $O_2^{\cdot-}$ can be converted to H_2O_2 and these ROSs can induce pathogen killing, structural cell-wall protein cross-linking, and expression of various genes to constitute a full-blown defense response. (*Modified from* Mehdy MC. Active oxygen species in plant defense against pathogens. Plant Physiol 1994;105;467–72; with permission.)

Polyclonal antibodies raised against human $p22^{phox}$, $p47^{phox}$, and $p67^{phox}$ have detected cross-reacting plant proteins of similar molecular sizes [75,76]. However, plant genes encoding any of these components have never been reported.

Oxidative stress and allergic inflammation

All aerobic organisms use O_2 in one form or another to generate energy requirements for various metabolic processes and to maintain cellular homeostasis. However, the high energy–generating aerobic metabolism comes at a cost. ROS are generated as byproducts of the oxidative metabolism, and cells neutralize them through various antioxidant defense mechanisms. When the delicate balance between ROS and antioxidants tips toward ROS, cellular components are damaged, resulting in various diseases involving practically every organ and system. ROS have been implicated in allergic disorders such as allergic rhinitis and atopic dermatitis [77–79].

In the respiratory system, NAD(P)H oxidase–generated ROS play an important role in physiologic processes such as airway and vasculature remodeling and O_2 sensing [80] at the same time excessive ROS play a key role in pathogenesis of allergic asthma and acute respiratory distress syndrome [81,82]. Exhaled H_2O_2 and nitric oxide (NO) are increased in patients who have allergic asthma compared with controls [83,84]. Also, the level of ROS in the airways is inversely correlated to the predicted forced expiratory volume in 1 second in patients who have asthma [85]. High levels of ROS are also encountered in the exacerbation of allergic asthma [86]. The direct effects of ROS on airway smooth muscle and mucin production are considered the mechanisms through which ROS induce and exacerbate allergic asthma [87,88]. ROS can inhibit β-adrenergic function in the airway smooth muscle cells and make them prone to acetylcholine-induced airway contraction [89,90].

Inflammatory cells such as macrophages, neutrophils, and eosinophils are considered the primary source of $O_2^{\cdot -}$ anions in the airways. Airway macrophages in patients who have asthma produce more $O_2^{\cdot -}$ than those of control subjects [91]. Even the monocytes and eosinophils collected from the blood of patients who have asthma produce more ROS compared with those of control subjects [91]. Environmental pollutants such as ozone, diesel exhaust, and cigarette smoke also increase $O_2^{\cdot -}$ production in the lungs and worsen the symptoms of allergic asthma [92–94]. These studies unraveled the important role of ROS in allergic airway inflammation, and considered inflammatory cell–generated and environmental ROS to be the major source. Many patients have sensitivity to plant pollens and develop allergic symptoms on exposure to the specific plant pollens. Plant tissues possess NADPH oxidase and generate ROS when activated. Intrigued by this observation, the authors sought to determine whether pollens contain NADPH oxidase and, if so, what role pollen NADPH oxidase plays in allergic airway inflammation.

Pollen NADPH oxidase in allergic inflammation

Pollens are complex biologic entities that deliver sperms to the ovule in flowering plants. For reproductive function, matured pollen must germinate a polarized pollen tube that grows toward the ovule. The process of pollen tube growth is highly structured and regulated by Rac homologs and Ca^{2+} signaling [95,96]. Because NAD(P)H oxidase is present in various plant tissues, and homologs of Rac2 are present in pollens and pollen tubes [97], the authors hypothesized that NAD(P)H oxidase components were present in plant pollens and discovered that many plant pollen extracts contain NADH/NAD(P)H-dependent oxidase activity [16]. The authors showed that ragweed and other pollen extracts reduce nitroblue tetrazolium chloride (NBT) to formazan in the presence of NAD(P)H (Fig. 6A). Ragweed preparations that lacked NAD(P)H oxidase, such as Amb a 1 and heat-treated Ragweed extract (RWE^H), did not reduce NBT (see Fig. 6A). The authors

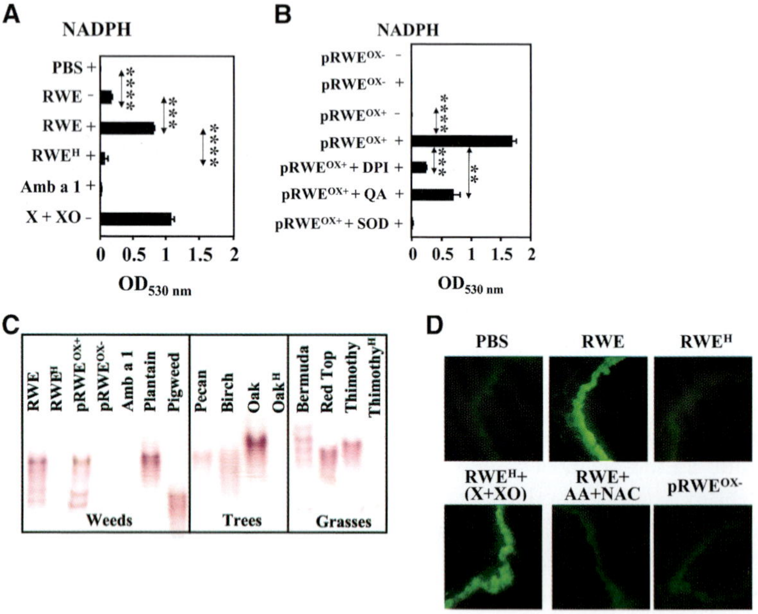

Fig. 6. Identification of pollen NAD(P)H oxidases. Plant pollen extracts possess NAD(P)H oxidase activity. (*A*) Reduction of NBT to formazan by allergenic extracts using NBT assay. RWE, RWE^H, and Amb a 1 were tested. X+XO was used as positive control. (*B*) $pRWE^{OX+}$–induced NBT reduction is inhibited by NAD(P)H oxidase inhibitors, DPI and quinacrine, and by the superoxide scavenger, SOD. (*C*) NBT reduction by allergenic extracts in situ after nondenaturing polyacrylamide gel electrophoresis. Oak^H, RWE^H, and $Timothy^H$ are heat-inactivated extracts. (*D*) Change in ROS levels in lung epithelium of mice after ex vivo challenge as determined through DCF fluorescence. (*Reproduced from* Boldogh I, Bacsi A, Choudhury BK, et al. ROS generated by pollen NAD(P)H oxidase provide a signal that augments antigen-induced allergic airway inflammation. J Clin Invest 2005;115(8):2169–79; with permission.)

fractionated RWE using size-exclusion chromatography and identified fractions that possessed or lacked NAD(P)H oxidase activity, termed $pRWE^{OX+}$ and $pRWE^{OX-}$. As hypothesized, $pRWE^{OX+}$, but not $pRWE^{OX-}$, reduced NBT in the presence of NAD(P)H (Fig. 6B). Adding NAD(P)H oxidase inhibitors DPI and quinacrine and the superoxide scavenger superoxide dismutase blocked this activity, suggesting the presence of NAD(P)H oxidase in the extracts. Furthermore, RWE also reduced redox-sensitive 2′-7′ dihydro-dichlorofluorescein diacetate (H_2 DCF-DA) into fluorescent DCF. These experiments suggested the generation of $O_2^{\cdot -}$ anions, which was confirmed through cytochrome C assay. In situ NBT gel assay on different pollen extract proteins after nondenaturing polyacrylamide gel electrophoresis showed well-defined protein bands only in the presence of NAD(P)H (Fig. 6C).

After the authors confirmed the presence of NAD(P)H oxidase in ragweed and other pollen extracts, they determined its role in allergic inflammation. They showed that RWE induces ROS in airway epithelial cells grown at the air–liquid interphase and in the murine airways (Fig. 6D). RWE^{H} and $pRWE^{OX-}$ resulted in minimal induction of ROS in either cells or the airways (see Fig. 6D). Using a murine model of allergic airway inflammation, the authors showed that RWE-induced inflammatory cell and eosinophil recruitment and mucin production were dependent on NAD(P)H oxidase activity of RWE (Fig. 7A–C), and observed a similar phenomenon in a murine model of allergic conjunctivitis. They proposed a two-signal model for the development of allergic inflammation, wherein signal 1 constitutes pollen NAD(P)H oxidase induced ROS and signal 2 is induced by antigen recognition through adaptive immune response. Both signals are required for robust allergic inflammation, and compromising either signal substantially reduces allergic process. Thus, pollen NAD(P)H oxidase–induced ROS plays a major role in allergic inflammatory processes in the airways and conjunctiva.

Summary

ROS are inevitable byproducts of various physiologic processes in the body. Maintenance of homeostatic balance between production of ROS and the mechanisms that scavenge ROS is a cornerstone of preventing pathogenesis of many diseases. Oxidative stress is the end result of numerous molecular pathways and mechanisms in which the endogenous antioxidant defenses yield to free radicals. Apart from known sources of ROS, pollen NAD(P)H oxidase constitutes an important enzyme contributing to asthma pathogenesis. Similar to mammalian cells, plants have developed sophisticated mechanisms for self-defense, including NAD(P)H oxidase–induced ROS. NAD(P)H oxidase has been identified in various plant species that is homologous to human $gp91^{phox}$. The NAD(P)H oxidase present in many plant tissues, including pollens, regulate various physiologic processes.

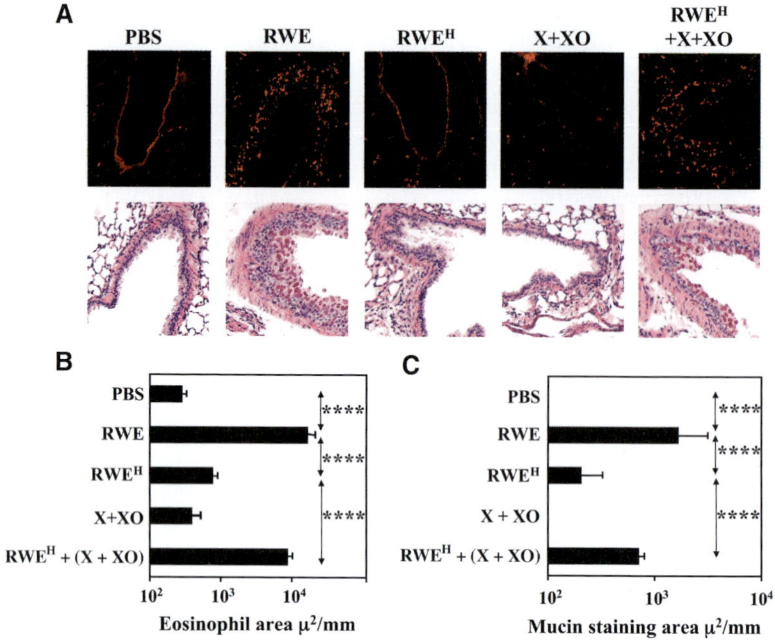

Fig. 7. ROS induced by NAD(P)H oxidase are required for allergic lung inflammation and mucin production. (*A*) Removal of NAD(P)H oxidase activity from RWE decreases accumulation of eosinophils in peribronchial location and mucin-containing cells in airway epithelium. Immunohistochemical staining of lung cryosections showing accumulation of eosinophils in peribronchial regions of lungs (*upper panel*). Periodic acid Schiff (PAS)–staining for mucin in representative lung sections (*lower panel*). Magenta-colored epithelial cells are positive for mucin. Magnification, 100X. (*B*) Total area of eosinophils in peribronchial area was quantified by morphometric analyses using Metamorph software. (*C*) Total area of mucin-containing cells in peribronchial area was quantified through morphometric analyses. Results are means ± s.e.m. (n = 7–9 mice per group). ***$P < .001$; ****$P < .0001$. (*Reproduced from* Boldogh I, Bacsi A, Choudhury BK, et al. ROS generated by pollen NAD(P)H oxidase provide a signal that augments antigen-induced allergic airway inflammation. J Clin Invest 2005;115(8):2169–79; with permission.)

The same NAD(P)H oxidase that provides an important defense mechanism for plants is detrimental to the cells lining the airways in humans when they generate ROS and perpetuate allergic airway inflammation. The authors identified an important mechanism through which plant pollens induce allergic inflammation in the lungs and conjunctiva, which is just a beginning in the new direction to understanding the molecular mechanisms of allergic inflammation. Much work needs to be done before the entire mechanistic pathway can be identified that is activated during exposure of airway cells to ROS. Although these studies would be very challenging because of the short half-life of the ROS, this area is worth exploring considering its ubiquitous presence in many human diseases.

Important questions and future directions

Currently, only one homolog of the human NAD(P)H oxidase is identified in plants. Plants likely posses other components similar to mammalian NAD(P)H oxidase, and the discovery of these will help experts understand in detail the process of ROS generation in plants. The signaling pathway in cells from the moment of their exposure to ROS to the end result (allergic inflammation) is still largely unknown. Identification of effects of ROS on genome-wide changes in the cells and its expression pattern will provide crucial links to current understanding. The effect of plant NAD(P)H oxidase on allergic airway inflammation in humans is not known. Therefore, studies should be conducted to answer these questions and devise therapeutic strategies to control pollen-induced allergic inflammation. Development of a newer generation of antioxidants that has a long biologic half-life at the local site would be of immense importance for treating allergic inflammation.

References

[1] Sedgwick JB, Vrtis RF, Gourley MF, et al. Stimulus-dependent differences in superoxide anion generation by normal human eosinophils and neutrophils. J Allergy Clin Immunol 1988;81(5 Pt 1):876–83.
[2] Creticos PS, Reed CE, Norman PS, et al. Ragweed immunotherapy in adult asthma. N Engl J Med 1996;334(8):501–7.
[3] Taylor PE, Flagan RC, Valenta R, et al. Release of allergens as respirable aerosols: a link between grass pollen and asthma. J Allergy Clin Immunol 2002;109(1):51–6.
[4] Walker SM, Pajno GB, Lima MT, et al. Grass pollen immunotherapy for seasonal rhinitis and asthma: a randomized, controlled trial. J Allergy Clin Immunol 2001;107(1):87–93.
[5] Gadermaier G, Dedic A, Obermeyer G, et al. Biology of weed pollen allergens. Curr Allergy Asthma Rep 2004;4(5):391–400.
[6] Doke N, Miura Y, Sanchez LM, et al. The oxidative burst protects plants against pathogen attack: mechanism and role as an emergency signal for plant bio-defence–a review. Gene 1996;179(1):45–51.
[7] Van Gestelen P, Asard H, Caubergs RJ. Solubilization and separation of a plant plasma membrane NADPH-O2- synthase from other NAD(P)H oxidoreductases. Plant Physiol 1997;115(2):543–50.
[8] Frahry G, Schopfer P. NADH-stimulated, cyanide-resistant superoxide production in maize coleoptiles analyzed with a tetrazolium-based assay. Planta 2001;212(2):175–83.
[9] Murphy TM, Vu H, Nguyen T. The superoxide synthases of rose cells. Comparison of assays. Plant Physiol 1998;117(4):1301–5.
[10] Wojtaszek P. Oxidative burst: an early plant response to pathogen infection. Biochem J 1997; 322(Pt 3):681–92.
[11] Yoshioka H, Sugie K, Park HJ, et al. Induction of plant gp91 phox homolog by fungal cell wall, arachidonic acid, and salicylic acid in potato. Mol Plant Microbe Interact 2001;14(6): 725–36.
[12] Sagi M, Fluhr R. Superoxide production by plant homologues of the gp91(phox) NADPH oxidase. Modulation of activity by calcium and by tobacco mosaic virus infection. Plant Physiol 2001;126(3):1281–90.
[13] Schopfer P, Plachy C, Frahry G. Release of reactive oxygen intermediates (superoxide radicals, hydrogen peroxide, and hydroxyl radicals) and peroxidase in germinating radish seeds controlled by light, gibberellin, and abscisic acid. Plant Physiol 2001;125(4):1591–602.

[14] Papadakis AK, Roubelakis-Angelakis KA. The generation of active oxygen species differs in tobacco and grapevine mesophyll protoplasts. Plant Physiol 1999;121(1):197–206.

[15] Foreman J, Demidchik V, Bothwell JH, et al. Reactive oxygen species produced by NADPH oxidase regulate plant cell growth. Nature 2003;422(6930):442–6.

[16] Boldogh I, Bacsi A, Choudhury BK, et al. ROS generated by pollen NADPH oxidase provide a signal that augments antigen-induced allergic airway inflammation. J Clin Invest 2005; 115(8):2169–79.

[17] Bulsior BM. Phagocytes of oxidative stress. Am J Med 2000;109:33–44.

[18] Baldridge CW, Gerard RW. The extra respiration of phagocytosis. Am J Physiol 1933;103: 235.

[19] Sbarra AJ, Karnovsky ML. The biochemical basis of phagocytosis. I. Metabolic changes during the ingestion of particles by polymorphonuclear leukocytes. J Biol Chem 1959; 234(6):1355–62.

[20] Selvaraj RJ, Sbarra AJ. Relationship of glycolytic and oxidative metabolism to particle entry and destruction in phagocytosing cells. Nature 1966;211(55):1272–6.

[21] Klebanoff S. A peroxidase-mediated antimicrobial system in leukocytes. J Clin Invest 1967; 46:1478–88.

[22] Holmes B, Page AR, Good RA. Studies of the metabolic activity of leukocytes from patients with a genetic abnormality of phagocytic function. J Clin Invest 1967;46(9):1422–32.

[23] McCord JM, Fridovich I. Superoxide dismutase. An enzymic function for erythrocuprein (hemocuprein). J Biol Chem 1969;244(22):6049–55.

[24] Hirata F, Hayaishi O. Possible participation of superoxide anion in the intestinal tryptophan 2,3-dioxygenase reaction. J Biol Chem 1971;246(24):7825–6.

[25] Strobel HW, Coon MJ. Effect of superoxide generation and dismutation on hydroxylation reactions catalyzed by liver microsomal cytochrome P-450. J Biol Chem 1971;246(24): 7826–9.

[26] Babior BM, Kipnes RS, Curnutte JT. Biological defense mechanisms. The production by leukocytes of superoxide, a potential bactericidal agent. J Clin Invest 1973;52(3):741–4.

[27] Batot G, Martel C, Capdeville N, et al. Characterization of neutrophil NADPH oxidase activity reconstituted in a cell-free assay using specific monoclonal antibodies raised against cytochrome b558. Eur J Biochem 1995;234(1):208–15.

[28] Bolscher BG, Koenderman L, Tool AT, et al. NADPH:O2 oxidoreductase of human eosinophils in the cell-free system. FEBS Lett 1990;268(1):269–73.

[29] Brozna JP, Hauff NF, Phillips WA, et al. Activation of the respiratory burst in macrophages. Phosphorylation specifically associated with Fc receptor-mediated stimulation. J Immunol 1988;141(5):1642–7.

[30] Volpp BD, Nauseef WM, Donelson JE, et al. Cloning of the cDNA and functional expression of the 47-kilodalton cytosolic component of human neutrophil respiratory burst oxidase. Proc Natl Acad Sci U S A 1989;86(18):7195–9.

[31] Volpp BD, Nauseef WM, Clark RA. Two cytosolic neutrophil oxidase components absent in autosomal chronic granulomatous disease. Science 1988;242(4883):1295–7.

[32] Leto TL, Lomax KJ, Volpp BD, et al. Cloning of a 67-kD neutrophil oxidase factor with similarity to a noncatalytic region of p60c-src. Science 1990;248(4956):727–30.

[33] Dinauer MC, Pierce EA, Bruns GA, et al. Human neutrophil cytochrome b light chain (p22-phox). Gene structure, chromosomal location, and mutations in cytochrome-negative autosomal recessive chronic granulomatous disease. J Clin Invest 1990;86(5): 1729–37.

[34] Clark RA, Volpp BD, Leidal KG, et al. Two cytosolic components of the human neutrophil respiratory burst oxidase translocate to the plasma membrane during cell activation. J Clin Invest 1990;85(3):714–21.

[35] Gabig TG, Crean CD, Mantel PL, et al. Function of wild-type or mutant Rac2 and Rap1a GTPases in differentiated HL60 cell NADPH oxidase activation. Blood 1995; 85(3):804–11.

[36] Ponting CP. Novel domains in NADPH oxidase subunits, sorting nexins, and PtdIns 3-kinases: binding partners of SH3 domains? Protein Sci 1996;5(11):2353–7.

[37] Kanai F, Liu H, Field SJ, et al. The PX domains of p47phox and p40phox bind to lipid products of PI(3)K. Nat Cell Biol 2001;3(7):675–8.

[38] Ago T, Nunoi H, Ito T, et al. Mechanism for phosphorylation-induced activation of the phagocyte NADPH oxidase protein p47(phox). Triple replacement of serines 303, 304, and 328 with aspartates disrupts the SH3 domain-mediated intramolecular interaction in p47(phox), thereby activating the oxidase. J Biol Chem 1999;274(47):33644–53.

[39] Gorlach A, Lee PL, Roesler J, et al. A p47-phox pseudogene carries the most common mutation causing p47-phox- deficient chronic granulomatous disease. J Clin Invest 1997; 100(8):1907–18.

[40] Noack D, Rae J, Cross AR, et al. Autosomal recessive chronic granulomatous disease caused by defects in NCF-1, the gene encoding the phagocyte p47-phox: mutations not arising in the NCF-1 pseudogenes. Blood 2001;97(1):305–11.

[41] Freeman JL, Lambeth JD. NADPH oxidase activity is independent of p47phox in vitro. J Biol Chem 1996;271(37):22578–82.

[42] Diekmann D, Abo A, Johnston C, et al. Interaction of Rac with p67phox and regulation of phagocytic NADPH oxidase activity. Science 1994;265(5171):531–3.

[43] Nisimoto Y, Motalebi S, Han CH, et al. The p67(phox) activation domain regulates electron flow from NADPH to flavin in flavocytochrome b(558). J Biol Chem 1999;274(33): 22999–3005.

[44] Han CH, Freeman JL, Lee T, et al. Regulation of the neutrophil respiratory burst oxidase. Identification of an activation domain in p67(phox). J Biol Chem 1998;273(27):16663–8.

[45] Ito T, Matsui Y, Ago T, et al. Novel modular domain PB1 recognizes PC motif to mediate functional protein-protein interactions. EMBO J 2001;20(15):3938–46.

[46] Polack B, Vergnaud S, Paclet MH, et al. Protein delivery by Pseudomonas type III secretion system: ex vivo complementation of p67(phox)-deficient chronic granulomatous disease-Biochem Biophys Res Commun 2000;275(3):854–8.

[47] Fuchs A, Dagher MC, Vignais PV. Mapping the domains of interaction of p40phox with both p47phox and p67phox of the neutrophil oxidase complex using the two-hybrid system. J Biol Chem 1995;270(11):5695–7.

[48] Kuribayashi F, Nunoi H, Wakamatsu K, et al. The adaptor protein p40(phox) as a positive regulator of the superoxide-producing phagocyte oxidase. EMBO J 2002;21(23):6312–20.

[49] Lopes LR, Dagher MC, Gutierrez A, et al. Phosphorylated p40PHOX as a negative regulator of NADPH oxidase. Biochemistry 2004;43(12):3723–30.

[50] Rotrosen D, Yeung CL, Leto TL, et al. Cytochrome b558: the flavin-binding component of the phagocyte NADPH oxidase. Science 1992;256(5062):1459–62.

[51] Roberts AW, Kim C, Zhen L, et al. Deficiency of the hematopoietic cell-specific Rho family GTPase Rac2 is characterized by abnormalities in neutrophil function and host defense. Immunity 1999;10(2):183–96.

[52] Abo A, Pick E, Hall A, et al. Activation of the NADPH oxidase involves the small GTP-binding protein p21rac1. Nature 1991;353(6345):668–70.

[53] Heyworth PG, Bohl BP, Bokoch GM, et al. Rac translocates independently of the neutrophil NADPH oxidase components p47phox and p67phox. Evidence for its interaction with flavocytochrome b558. J Biol Chem 1994;269(49):30749–52.

[54] Cross AR, Heyworth PG, Rae J, et al. A variant X-linked chronic granulomatous disease patient (X91+) with partially functional cytochrome b. J Biol Chem 1995; 270(14):8194–200.

[55] Ambruso DR, Knall C, Abell AN, et al. Human neutrophil immunodeficiency syndrome is associated with an inhibitory Rac2 mutation. Proc Natl Acad Sci U S A 2000;97(9):4654–9.

[56] Henderson LM, Chappell JB, Jones OT. Internal pH changes associated with the activity of NADPH oxidase of human neutrophils. Further evidence for the presence of an H+ conducting channel. Biochem J 1988;251(2):563–7.

[57] Kaneda M, Sakuraba H, Ohtake A, et al. Missense mutations in the gp91-phox gene encoding cytochrome b558 in patients with cytochrome b positive and negative X-linked chronic granulomatous disease. Blood 1999;93(6):2098–104.
[58] Pollock JD, Williams DA, Gifford MA, et al. Mouse model of X-linked chronic granulomatous disease, an inherited defect in phagocyte superoxide production. Nat Genet 1995;9(2): 202–9.
[59] Yu L, Zhen L, Dinauer MC. Biosynthesis of the phagocyte NADPH oxidase cytochrome b558. Role of heme incorporation and heterodimer formation in maturation and stability of gp91phox and p22phox subunits. J Biol Chem 1997;272(43):27288–94.
[60] Porter CD, Parkar MH, Verhoeven AJ, et al. p22-phox-deficient chronic granulomatous disease: reconstitution by retrovirus-mediated expression and identification of a biosynthetic intermediate of gp91-phox. Blood 1994;84(8):2767–75.
[61] Fath A, Bethke P, Beligni V, et al. Active oxygen and cell death in cereal aleurone cells. J Exp Bot 2002;53(372):1273–82.
[62] Pei ZM, Murata Y, Benning G, et al. Calcium channels activated by hydrogen peroxide mediate abscisic acid signalling in guard cells. Nature 2000;406(6797):731–4.
[63] Joo JH, Bae YS, Lee JS. Role of auxin-induced reactive oxygen species in root gravitropism. Plant Physiol 2001;126(3):1055–60.
[64] Bais HP, Vepachedu R, Gilroy S, et al. Allelopathy and exotic plant invasion: from molecules and genes to species interactions. Science 2003;301(5638):1377–80.
[65] Doke N. Generation of superoxide anion by potato tuber protoplasts during the hypersensitive response to hyphal cell wall components of Phytophthora infestans and specific inhibition of the reaction by suppressors of hypersensitivity. Physiol Plant Pathol 1983;23:359–67.
[66] Jabs T, Tschope M, Colling C, et al. Elicitor-stimulated ion fluxes and O2- from the oxidative burst are essential components in triggering defense gene activation and phytoalexin synthesis in parsley. Proc Natl Acad Sci U S A 1997;94(9):4800–5.
[67] Doke N, Miura Y. In vitro activation of NADPH-dependent O_2- generating system in a plasma membrane-rich fraction of potato tuber tissues by treatment with an elicitor from Phytophthora infestans or with digitonin. Physiol Plant Pathol 1995;46:17–28.
[68] Groom QJ, Torres MA, Fordham-Skelton AP, et al. RbohA, a rice homologue of the mammalian gp91phox respiratory burst oxidase gene. Plant J 1996;10(3):515–22.
[69] Torres MA, Onouchi H, Hamada S, et al. Six Arabidopsis thaliana homologues of the human respiratory burst oxidase (gp91phox). Plant J 1998;14(3):365–70.
[70] Amicucci EGK, Ward JM. NADPH oxidase genes from tomato (Lycopersicon esculentum) and curly-leaf pondweed (Potamogeton crispus). Plant Biol 1999;1:524–8.
[71] Yoshioka H, Numata N, Nakajima K, et al. Nicotiana benthamiana gp91phox homologs NbrbohA and NbrbohB participate in H2O2 accumulation and resistance to Phytophthora infestans. Plant Cell 2003;15(3):706–18.
[72] Berken A, Thomas C, Wittinghofer A. A new family of RhoGEFs activates the Rop molecular switch in plants. Nature 2005;436(7054):1176–80.
[73] Ono E, Wong HL, Kawasaki T, et al. Essential role of the small GTPase Rac in disease resistance of rice. Proc Natl Acad Sci U S A 2001;98(2):759–64.
[74] Morel J, Fromentin J, Blein JP, et al. Rac regulation of NtrbohD, the oxidase responsible for the oxidative burst in elicited tobacco cell. Plant J 2004;37(2):282–93.
[75] Desikan R, Hancock JT, Coffey MJ, et al. Generation of active oxygen in elicited cells of Arabidopsis thaliana is mediated by a NADPH oxidase-like enzyme. FEBS Lett 1996; 382(1–2):213–7.
[76] Tenhaken R, Levine A, Brisson LF, et al. Function of the oxidative burst in hypersensitive disease resistance. Proc Natl Acad Sci U S A 1995;92(10):4158–63.
[77] Iijima MK, Kobayashi T, Kamada H, et al. Exposure to ozone aggravates nasal allergy-like symptoms in guinea pigs. Toxicol Lett 2001;123(1):77–85.
[78] Polla BS, Ezekowitz RA, Leung DY. Monocytes from patients with atopic dermatitis are primed for superoxide production. J Allergy Clin Immunol 1992;89(2):545–51.

[79] Briganti S, Cristaudo A, D'Argento V, et al. Oxidative stress in physical urticarias. Clin Exp Dermatol 2001;26(3):284–8.
[80] Hoidal JR, Brar SS, Sturrock AB, et al. The role of endogenous NADPH oxidases in airway and pulmonary vascular smooth muscle function. Antioxid Redox Signal 2003;5(6):751–8.
[81] Vachier I, Damon M, Le Doucen C, et al. Increased oxygen species generation in blood monocytes of asthmatic patients. Am Rev Respir Dis 1992;146(5 Pt 1):1161–6.
[82] Moraes TJ, Zurawska JH, Downey GP. Neutrophil granule contents in the pathogenesis of lung injury. Curr Opin Hematol 2006;13(1):21–7.
[83] Emelyanov A, Fedoseev G, Abulimity A, et al. Elevated concentrations of exhaled hydrogen peroxide in asthmatic patients. Chest 2001;120(4):1136–9.
[84] Ganas K, Loukides S, Papatheodorou G, et al. Total nitrite/nitrate in expired breath condensate of patients with asthma. Respir Med 2001;95(8):649–54.
[85] Jarjour NN, Calhoun WJ. Enhanced production of oxygen radicals in asthma. J Lab Clin Med 1994;123(1):131–6.
[86] Mak JC, Leung HC, Ho SP, et al. Systemic oxidative and antioxidative status in Chinese patients with asthma. J Allergy Clin Immunol 2004;114(2):260–4.
[87] Stewart RM, Weir EK, Montgomery MR, et al. Hydrogen peroxide contracts airway smooth muscle: a possible endogenous mechanism. Respir Physiol 1981;45(3):333–42.
[88] Wright DT, Fischer BM, Li C, et al. Oxidant stress stimulates mucin secretion and PLC in airway epithelium via a nitric oxide-dependent mechanism. Am J Physiol 1996;271(5 Pt 1): L854–61.
[89] Nijkamp FP, Henricks PA. Receptors in airway disease. Beta-adrenoceptors in lung inflammation. Am Rev Respir Dis 1990;141(3 Pt 2):S145–50.
[90] Katsumata U, Miura M, Ichinose M, et al. Oxygen radicals produce airway constriction and hyperresponsiveness in anesthetized cats. Am Rev Respir Dis 1990;141(5 Pt 1):1158–61.
[91] Calhoun WJ, Reed HE, Moest DR, et al. Enhanced superoxide production by alveolar macrophages and air-space cells, airway inflammation, and alveolar macrophage density changes after segmental antigen bronchoprovocation in allergic subjects. Am Rev Respir Dis 1992;145(2 Pt 1):317–25.
[92] Comhair SA, Thomassen MJ, Erzurum SC. Differential induction of extracellular glutathione peroxidase and nitric oxide synthase 2 in airways of healthy individuals exposed to 100% O(2) or cigarette smoke. Am J Respir Cell Mol Biol 2000;23(3):350–4.
[93] Jung M, Davis WP, Taatjes DJ, et al. Asbestos and cigarette smoke cause increased DNA strand breaks and necrosis in bronchiolar epithelial cells in vivo. Free Radic Biol Med 2000;28(8):1295–9.
[94] Michalec L, Choudhury BK, Postlethwait E, et al. CCL7 and CXCL10 orchestrate oxidative stress-induced neutrophilic lung inflammation. J Immunol 2002;168(2):846–52.
[95] Kost B, Lemichez E, Spielhofer P, et al. Rac homologues and compartmentalized phosphatidylinositol 4, 5-bisphosphate act in a common pathway to regulate polar pollen tube growth. J Cell Biol 1999;145(2):317–30.
[96] Pierson ES, Miller DD, Callaham DA, et al. Tip-localized calcium entry fluctuates during pollen tube growth. Dev Biol 1996;174(1):160–73.
[97] Lin Y, Yang Z. Inhibition of pollen tube elongation by microinjected Anti-Rop1Ps antibodies suggests a crucial role for Rho-type GTPases in the control of tip growth. Plant Cell 1997;9(9):1647–59.

ELSEVIER
SAUNDERS

Immunol Allergy Clin N Am
27 (2007) 65–78

IMMUNOLOGY
AND ALLERGY
CLINICS
OF NORTH AMERICA

Impact of Native, Recombinant, and Cross-Reactive Allergens on Humoral and T-Cell–Mediated Immune Responses

Reto Crameri, PhD[a,b,*], Claudio Rhyner, PhD[a]

[a]*Division of Molecular Allergology, Swiss Institute of Allergy and Asthma Research (SIAF), Obere Strasse 22, CH-7270 Davos, Switzerland*
[b]*Department of Molecular Biology, University of Salzburg, Hellbrunnerstrasse 34, A-5020 Austria*

Allergic and asthmatic diseases are an increasing health burden affecting large parts of the population, and the incidence of the diseases is still increasing [1,2]. T-cell responses to allergens are the key regulators of the pathogenesis of allergic disease, such as rhinitis, conjunctivitis, atopic dermatitis, and bronchial asthma, and allergic responses to insect stings and food ingestion [3,4]. The disease complex is an important cause of morbidity and, occasionally, mortality [5]. Therapeutic approaches to control allergy and asthma include symptomatic treatment with antihistamines, corticosteroids, bronchodilators (β-adrenergic receptor antagonists), and anti-IgE antibody therapy [6,7]. These drugs ameliorate allergy symptoms and concomitant inflammatory reactions, but require long-term recurrent administration [8].

Therefore, until primary prevention succeeds, immunomodulation will remain the principal practical approach to controlling allergic diseases. Allergen-specific immunotherapy (SIT), introduced in early twentieth century, is the only treatment that can cure allergic diseases [9,10]. Despite considerable success in individuals sensitized to insect venom [11] and pollen-mediated allergy [12], the clinical benefits in treating more complex allergy forms, such as those to house dust mites, mold, or food, are disappointing and largely contradictory. These limitations might be caused by factors related

This work was supported by Grants No. 31-63382.00/2 and 310000-114634/1 from the Swiss National Science Foundation and by the OPO-Pharma Foundation, Zürich.

* Corresponding author. Division of Molecular Allergology, Swiss Institute of Allergy and Asthma Research (SIAF), Obere Strasse 22, CH-7270 Davos, Switzerland.

E-mail address: crameri@siaf.unizh.ch (R. Crameri).

doi:10.1016/j.iac.2006.11.003

to the type of adjuvant, route of application, and duration of treatment used. However, the most important reason for SIT failure probably relates to the type of vaccine used, although confirmatory studies for this assumption are lacking.

Although insect venoms and pollen extracts are easily standardized, extracts from complex allergen sources, such as mites, molds, and foods, which contain dozens of structurally different allergen molecules [13–15], are difficult to standardize [16]. The best example is represented by commercially available mold extracts that contain major allergens in concentrations varying over three orders of magnitude [17]. Using these extracts in SIT and studies investigating the mechanisms underlying immunotherapy, which are both concentration-dependent, obviously cannot be expected to deliver reproducible results when different batches of a given extract are used. Using biochemically purified natural allergens or recombinant allergens, which are standardized in absolute terms through physicochemical methods, will contribute to a detailed understanding of the immunologic mechanisms underlying the pathology of type I hypersensitivity reactions. Progress in understanding the mechanisms governing SIT will help experts generate ideas and concepts for improving therapeutic schedules and provide a scientifically based, reproducible, and safe treatment for allergic disease.

Native and recombinant allergens

Although older literature and current allergology practice define *allergen* as an extract from a natural allergen source [18,19], molecular biologists define it as a single molecular structure able to bind IgE from sera of individuals sensitized to that particular molecule. This difference in definition has far-reaching consequences for basic experiments, diagnosis, and treatment of allergic diseases. Every experimental or clinical setup involving allergen extracts depends on the quality of the extract used, which strongly depends on the batch used [20,21] and the heterogenous, polyclonal responses to natural exposure that elicit patient-specific IgE responses to a variable pattern of allergen structures present in the extract [22,23]. This unlucky situation does not allow patient stratification, and does not permit experts to know a priori either the number of molecular structures to which a given patient is sensitized or if the extract contains the single allergens in sufficient amounts to obtain the desired diagnostic or therapeutic effect. In fact, increasing clinical evidence shows that SIT can induce sensitization to molecular allergen structures to which the patients were not allergic before treatment [24,25].

The application of biochemical methods to purify single allergens from complex extracts [26,27] and the introduction of molecular biology techniques in allergology research [28–34] have drastically changed this picture. This fact is best exemplified by phospholipase A_2 (PLA_2), a major allergen of bee venom (Api m 1), which has been available as biochemically purified protein from the natural source for decades and was later cloned and produced as recombinant allergen [35]. The availability of both native and recombinant PLA_2 allowed experts to show that allergens can be produced as highly pure recombinant proteins in an active form with biochemical and immunologic properties practically indistinguishable from those of their native counterparts [35]. Natural and recombinant PLA_2 have been shown to have comparable type I skin reactivity [36] and the same potency to release histamine from basophiles [37]. Moreover, the structure [38], but not the enzymatic activity [39], could be shown to be important for the immunogenicity of the protein. Recombinant PLA_2 also has been shown to be useful in increasing the specificity of diagnostic tests [40], a property that seems to be typical for recombinant allergens [15,41–44]. Recombinant allergens can easily be used in fully automated diagnostic devices [45,46]. Recombinant allergens can be produced as standardized proteins with biochemical properties practically indistinguishable from those of natural allergens and of a quality that satisfies the standards for use in humans. They will most likely replace most extracts for diagnosing allergic conditions in the near future.

The most important issue, however, is that recombinant allergens have drastically changed the understanding of allergy, opening frontiers for the development of new diagnostic and therapeutic concepts. Based on a long list of cloned allergens [47], it is now possible, at last in specialized research laboratories, to determine patient-specific sensitization profiles and thus to perform a component-resolved diagnosis of allergy [48]. The ability to stratify patients according to the molecular structures responsible for the patient-specific sensitization will allow the possibility of patient-tailored, component resolved immunotherapy in the future [49].

Purified native and recombinant allergens have strongly contributed to expanding the knowledge of the basic mechanisms modulating the immune response against normally innocuous environmental antigens and allergens in healthy and allergic individuals. Native and recombinant bee venom PLA_2 have played a pivotal role in modern allergology, and work performed at T-cell level with these substances has strongly influenced this field. Most individuals stung by a bee initially elicit low-affinity IgG1 anti-PLA_2 antibodies and develop high-affinity IgG4 antibodies to PLA_2 after repeated exposure [50]. In contrast, some individuals generate PLA_2-specific IgE antibodies and develop bee sting allergy [51]. PLA_2 displays three immunodominant T-cell epitopes (Fig. 1) equally recognized by allergic and nonallergic individuals [52], and one glycopeptide T-cell recognition site [53]. These epitopes are equally recognized by allergic and nonallergic individuals [54] and have been successfully used in specific immunotherapy of patients allergic to bee venom [55].

Cross-reactive allergens

Cross-reactive allergens represent the most interesting, but also the most challenging, molecular structures. The elucidation of hundreds of sequences

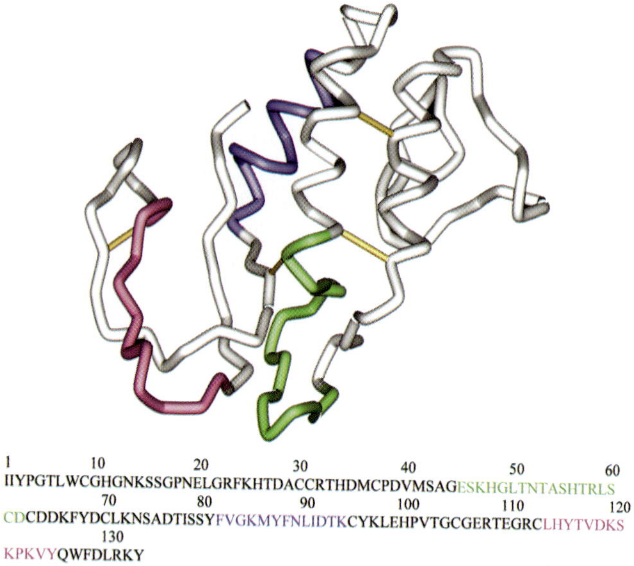

Fig. 1. Localization of the linear T-cell epitopes of PLA_2, the major bee venom allergen, on the amino acid sequence and on the structure of the enzyme. The epitopes defined in T-cell proliferation experiments with overlapping peptides [52], highlighted in green, blue, and magenta in the linear structure, are depicted in the same colors on the three-dimensional context.

encoding allergens, combined with homology searches, enabled a first in silico identification of molecular families of homologous allergens potentially involved in cross-reactivity [56]. Bioinformatic analyses based on structural motifs [57], and Basic Local Alignment Search Tool (BLAST) similarity search methods [58] involving 1,01,602 and 1,35,850 protein entries deposited in the Swissprot database, predict 4093 (4%) and 4768 (3.5%) different potential allergen structures, respectively. Therefore, the allergen repertoire involved in eliciting allergic symptoms can be assumed to involve approximately 10^4 different molecules organized in a limited number of phylogenetically related families. The molecular basis underlying cross-reactivity is schematically represented in Fig. 2.

However, not all structures will be required for diagnostic and therapeutic applications because many allergens can be grouped in pan-allergen families sharing cross-reactive epitopes [59–63]. Cross-reactivity will help drastically reduce the number of epitopes needed for a careful diagnosis of allergy, and the rapidly increasing knowledge about primary and three-dimensional structures of allergens [56] will speed up theoretical and practical progress in defining the number of structures or epitopes needed for a component-resolved diagnosis of allergic diseases that forms the basis for the development of rational therapy approaches.

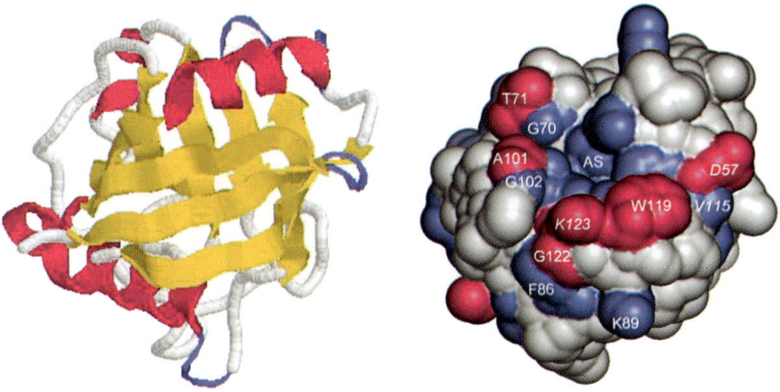

Fig. 2. Cross-reactivity derives from conserved amino acids exposed to the surface of molecules sharing extended homology at primary and tertiary structure. The left panel shows the overall fold of cyclophilin consisting of a central eight-stranded β-sheet (*yellow*) and two flanking α-helices (*pink*). The right panel shows a typical patch of the identical solvent-exposed amino acids (pink >50%, blue >30% exposed) deriving from the superposition of the *Malassezia Sympodialis* and human thioredoxin crystal structures. These amino acids located in different loops are assembled on the surface forming a potential conformational IgE-binding B-cell epitope. (*Adapted from* Limacher A, Glaser AG, Meier C, et al. Cross-reactivity and 1.4 Å crystal structure of *Malassezia sympodialis* Thioredoxin (Mala s 13), a member of a new pan-allergen family. J Immunol 2007;178:389–96.)

Humoral and T-cell mediated immune responses to cross-reactive structures

Studies have shown that recombinant allergens can be produced as perfectly standardized molecules with characteristics practically indistinguishable from those of their natural counterparts. The best documented examples are PLA_2, the major bee venom allergen [35], and Bet v 1, the major birch pollen allergen [64]. In vitro these recombinant allergens show IgE-binding capacity [42,65], potency to release mediators from effector cells [37,65], and potency to stimulate T-cell proliferation [52,64] comparable to those of the biochemically purified allergens from the natural source. Most importantly, the skin-test reactivity in vivo is no different between recombinant and natural allergens [36,42,43], definitively showing that recombinant allergens can substitute natural allergens for the in vitro and in vivo diagnosis of allergy. The list of recombinant allergens shown to be equivalent to their natural counterparts is long [66] and still growing rapidly. Again, Bet v 1 represents the best-characterized prototype of a cross-reactive structure present in many allergen sources, such as celery [67], apple [68], hazelnut [69], cherry [70], and carrot [41,71].

A special case of cross-reactive structures are defined by proteins showing IgE-mediated autoreactivity (Table 1) [72–80]. Increasing evidence shows that self antigens can induce IgE-mediated allergic responses. Therefore, experts must distinguish between indirect evidence obtained in in vitro

Table 1
Human proteins showing cross-reactivity with environmental allergens

Human protein	Molecular weight (kd)	Acc. no.	Cross-reactive with	Source	Reference
MnSOD	24.7	P04179	Asp f 6	*Aspergillus fumigatus*	[86]
			Dro m MnSOD	Fruit fly	[86]
			Hev b10	Latex	[72]
			Mala s 11	*Malassezia sympodialis*	[73]
			Sac c MnSOD	Baker's yeast	[86]
Profilin	14.9	P07737	Ara t 8	*Arabidopsis thaliana*	[74]
			Bet v 2	Birch	[75]
Cyclophilins (A/B/C)	17.8–22.7	P62937	Asp f 11	*Aspergillus fumigatus*	[86]
		P23284	Cand a CyP	*Candida albicans*	[86]
		P45877	Mala s 6	*Malassezia sympodialis*	[86]
			Sac c CyP	Baker's yeast	[86]
Thioredoxin	11.7	X77584	Tri a 25	Wheat	[94]
			Zea m 25	Corn	[94]
			Mala s 13	*Malassezia sympodialis*	[63]
Ribosomal protein P2	11.6	M17887	Alt a 5	*Alternaria alternata*	[90]
			Asp f 8	*Aspergillus fumigatus*	[90]
			Cla h 5	*Cladosporium herbarum*	[90]
APDH	—	—	Gad c APDH	Codfish	[76]
Casein	25.4	X17070	Bos d 8	Cow's milk	[77]
Lactalbumin	16.2	J00270	Bos d 4	Cow's milk	[78]
Insulin	12.0	V00565	Bos d insulin	Bovine insulin	[79]
			Sus s insulin	Porcine insulin	
Serum albumin	69.4	V00494	Bos d 6	Bovine serum albumin	[80]
			Can f 3	Canine serum albumin	
			Fel d 2	Feline serum albumin	
			Equ c 3	Equine serum albumin	

Abbreviations: Acc., accession; APDH, aldehyde phosphate dehydrogenase; MnSOD, manganese–dependant superoxide dismutase.

experiments or ex vivo experiments using isolated cells and direct evidence obtained from testing the self antigens in patients. Structurally, experts must distinguish between self antigens that have strong sequence identity, homology, and epitope mimicry to environmental allergens, and those that do not.

Besides profilin, which was the first self allergen shown to bind IgE from birch-sensitized patients in vitro [59], arrays of self antigens able to bind IgE isolated through different screening procedures also have been identified [81–83]. The first self antigen directly shown to induce type I skin reactions in patients was human manganese–dependant superoxide dismutase (MnSOD), a phylogenetically highly conserved protein [84]. This study showed that human MnSOD shares 51.5% identity and 67.2% homology with the corresponding allergen of *Aspergillus fumigatus* [85]. The two recombinant MnSODs were recognized by IgE antibodies from patients allergic to *A fumigatus* MnSOD, elicited specific type I reactions in these individuals, and induced specific proliferation of peripheral blood mononuclear cells from individuals allergic to *A fumigatus* who showed specific IgE responses and reacted in skin tests to MnSOD. Further studies showed that even MnSOD of *Drosophila melanogaster*, wherein exposure in the normal population can be virtually excluded, is able to bind IgE and induce T-cell proliferation in ex vivo material of individuals sensitized to MnSOD, indicating molecular mimicry is a basic mechanism for the observed reactivity [86]. Detailed comparisons of the crystal structures of human and *A fumigatus* MnSOD [87] and molecular modelling of additional MnSODs [86] allowed an exact definition of the potential amino acids defining cross-reactivity. Furthermore, studies have shown that human MnSOD directly applied to the skin of patients who have atopic eczema and are sensitized to *Malassezia sympodialis* in atopy patch tests is sufficient to elicit an eczematous reaction [88,89]. In concordance with the presence of MnSOD-specific IgE antibodies, determined using enzyme-linked immunosorbent assay (ELISA), the human enzyme also elicited positive skin test reactions in all patients who had positive ELISA results, and reactivity against human MnSOD strongly correlated with the severity of the disease, corroborating a pathogenic role of self-reactivity in the exacerbation of atopic eczema. However, MnSOD is not an exotic example because comparable patterns of autoreactivity also have been obtained with acidic ribosomal P_2 protein [90], cyclophilin [62,91,92], and thioredoxin [63]. Cyclophilin and thioredoxin were first identified as allergens through screening of phage-surface displayed libraries with sera of patients who had long-lasting atopic diseases [14,62]. The corresponding human enzymes were amplified from human cDNA libraries with polymerase chain reaction and used to produce the recombinant proteins [62,63]. Screening of the protein repertoires of wheat and maize with sera from patients who had positive results from a double-blind, placebo-controlled food challenge yielded, among the allergens cloned, thioredoxin as an additional allergenic structure [93]. The recombinant maize and wheat proteins displayed enzymatic activity, and bakers who had occupational asthma and patients who had grass pollen allergy but no clinical history of cereal allergy had sensitization rates of 47% and 35%, respectively [94]. The maize and wheat thioredoxins, sharing 74% sequence identity, exhibited distinct IgE cross-reactivity and also cross-reactivity to human thioredoxin.

As a first step in investigating cross-reactivity between cyclophilins and thioredoxins, the authors solved the crystal structures of *Malassezia sympodialis* cyclophilin [92] and thioredoxin [63]. Comparing these structures with the solved structures of human cyclophilin and thioredoxin allowed an exact definition of conserved amino acids exposed to the solvent that forms structural patches, potentially defining cross-reactive B-cell epitopes [63,92], as exemplified in Fig. 2. Although the authenticity of the postulated B-cell epitopes must be confirmed through site-directed mutagenesis, this will require crystallization and structure elucidation of each single mutant to confirm that the mutations do not affect the three-dimensional structure. Studies have shown that IgE binding exquisitely depends on the three-dimensional structure of the allergen [95,96], and therefore reduction of IgE binding through site-directed mutagenesis could be caused by either direct involvement of an amino acid exchanged at IgE binding or changes in the three-dimensional structure from the exchange without contribution of the changed amino acid to IgE binding. This crucial point is often neglected in site-directed mutagenesis experiments.

However, the list of self antigens involved in IgE binding is rapidly increasing, and autoreactivity clearly plays a role in the exacerbation of long-lasting atopic diseases [86,88–90,97]. Evidence comes from the ability of self antigens to induce strong humoral and T-cell–mediated reactions ex vivo, and from the ability of the self antigens to induce skin- and atopy patch test reactions in sensitized individuals [88,89]. Whether self antigens themselves are promoting the onset of IgE-mediated autoimmune reactions remains unclear. For self antigens sharing extended sequence identity or homology to environmental allergens, one can assume that autoreactivity is caused by molecular epitope mimicry at the B- and T-cell level [85,88,90]. For self antigens lacking significant sequence homology to environmental allergens, one cannot exclude that homologous, currently unidentified structures could be present in the incomplete repertoire of environmental proteins able to induce IgE sensitization. The available observations support the assumption that autoreactivity is initiated or at least preceded by a sensitization against environmental allergens [97]. If a human protein is available to the immune system, it will probably induce immune tolerance. However, this tolerance can be eluded through cross-reacting IgE antibodies raised against epitopes shared between human proteins and environmental allergens [98]. Although molecular mimicry between conserved T- and B-cell epitopes seems to be the most likely explanation for the observed autoimmune reactions to self antigens, more work remains to clarify if sensitization to self antigens can occur as a direct consequence of inflammatory processes.

Summary

Biochemical and molecular biology methods allow the production and purification of virtually pure natural and recombinant allergens. For the first time, immune responses to allergens could be dissected at the molecular level using pure reagents. Given that T-cell responses, which are the key regulators of atopic diseases, are highly dose-dependent and that doses can affect cytokine profiles, molecular characterization of natural, recombinant, and cross-reactive allergens realized an unmet experimental need. "Clean" and straightforward experimental setups using pure allergens allowed experts to clarify most of the contradictory results obtained using allergen extracts. Diagnostic procedures based on purified allergens have contributed to increasing specificity and sensitivity and determining patient-specific sensitization patterns. This stratification will allow development of patient-tailored therapeutic schedules, with defined allergen doses likely contributing to improving therapeutic effects. However, a breakthrough in specific therapy of allergy and asthma will depend on developing an understanding of the immunologic mechanisms underlying the diseases. Specific elimination of pathogenic T-cell subsets and targeted elimination of allergen-specific B cells seem the most promising approaches. Both strategies will require engineering of chimeric molecules able to cross-link receptors on the surface of targeted effector cells, and recombinant allergens will confer an absolute specificity to these novel therapeutic lead compounds.

References

[1] Bachau V, Durham SR. Prevalence and rate of diagnosis of allergic rhinitis in Europe. Eur Respir J 2004;24(5):758–64.
[2] Sennhauser FH, Braun-Fahrlander C, Wildhaber JH. The burden of asthma in children: a European perspective. Paediatr Respir Rev 2005;6(1):2–7.
[3] Kay AB. Allergy and allergic diseases. First of two parts. N Engl J Med 2001;344(1):30–7.
[4] Kay AB. Allergy and allergic diseases. Second of two parts. N Engl J Med 2001;344(2):109–13.
[5] Montanaro A, Bardana EJ Jr. The mechanisms, causes, and treatment of anaphylaxis. J Investig Allergol Clin Immunol 2002;12(1):2–11.
[6] Barnes PJ. Therapeutic strategies for allergic diseases. Nature 1999;402(Suppl 6760):B31–8.
[7] Strunk RC, Bloomberg GR. Omalizumab for asthma. N Engl J Med 2006;354(25):2689–95.
[8] Kankaanranta H, Lahdensuo A, Moilanen E, et al. Add-on therapy options in asthma not adequately controlled by inhaled corticosteroids: a comprehensive review. Respir Res 2004;5(1):17.
[9] Mascarell L, Van Overtvelt V, Moingeon P. Novel ways for immune intervention in immunotherapy: mucosal allergy vaccines. Immunol Allergy Clin North Am 2006;26:283–306.
[10] Noon L. Prophylactic inoculation against hay fever. Lancet 1911;1:1572–3.
[11] Müller UR. Bee venom allergy in beekeepers and their family members. Curr Opin Allergy Clin Immunol 2005;5(4):343–7.

[12] Durham SR, Walker SM, Varga EM, et al. Long-term clinical efficacy of grass-pollen immunotherapy. N Engl J Med 1999;341(7):468–75.
[13] Thomas WR, Smith W. Towards defining the full spectrum of important house dust mite allergens. Clin Exp Allergy 1999;29(12):896–904.
[14] Crameri R, Limacher A, Weichel M, et al. Structural aspects and clinical relevance of *Aspergillus fumigatus* antigens/allergens. Med Mycol 2006;44:S261–7.
[15] Bohle B, Vieths S. Improving diagnostic tests for food allergy with recombinant allergens. Methods 2003;32(3):292–9.
[16] van Ree R. The CREATE project: EU support for the improvement of allergen standardization in Europe. Allergy 2004;59(6):571–4.
[17] Vailes L, Sridhara S, Cromwell O, et al. Quantitation of the major fungal allergens, Alt a 1 and Asp f 1, in commercial allergenic products. J Allergy Clin Immunol 2001;107(4):641–6.
[18] Meinert R, Frischer T, Karmaus W, et al. Influence of skin prick test criteria on estimation of prevalence and incidence of allergic sensitization in children. Allergy 1994;49(7):526–32.
[19] Pastorello EA, Incorvaia C, Ortolani C, et al. Studies on the relationship between the level of specific IgE antibodies and the clinical expression of allergy: I. Definition of levels distinguishing patients with symptomatic from patients with asymptomatic allergy to common aeroallergens. J Allergy Clin Immunol 1995;96(5):580–7.
[20] Dreborg S. The batch-to-batch variationof the potency of dog- and cat- allergen-coated lancets. Evaluation by skin prick testing. Allergy 1993;48(5):373–6.
[21] Platts-Mills TAE, Chapman MD. Allergen standardization. J Allergy Clin Immunol 1991; 87:621–5.
[22] Muguerzat J, Capo C, Porri F, et al. Latex allergy: allergen identification in *Hevea brasiliensis* fractions by immunoblotting. Clin Exp Allergy 1996;26(10):1177–81.
[23] Lewis SA, Grimshaw KE, Warner JO, et al. The promiscuity of immunoglobulin E binding to peanut allergens, as determined by Western blotting, correlates with the severity of clinical symptoms. Clin Exp Allergy 2005;35(6):767–73.
[24] van Hage-Hamsten M, Valenta R. Specific immunotherapy—the induction of new IgE-specificities? Allergy 2002;57(5):375–8.
[25] Moverare R, Elfman L, Vesterinen E, et al. Development of new IgE specificities to allergic components in birch pollen extract during specific immunotherapy studied with immunoblotting and Pharmacia CAP System. Allergy 2002;57(5):423–30.
[26] Arruda LK, Platts-Mills TA, Fox JW, et al. *Aspergillus fumigatus* allergen I, a major IgE-binding protein, is a member of the mitogillin family of cytotoxins. J Exp Med 1990; 172(5):1529–32.
[27] Di Felice G, Tinghino R, Federico R, et al. Use of monoclonal antibodies for the characterization of allergenic extracts. Ann Ist Super Sanita 1991;27(1):183–7.
[28] Chua KY, Stewart GA, Thomas WR, et al. Sequence analysis of cDNA coding for a major house dust mite allergen, Der p 1. Homology with cysteine proteases. J Exp Med 1988;167(1): 175–82.
[29] Scheiner O. Recombinant allergens: biological, immunological and practical aspects. Int Arch Allergy Immunol 1992;98(2):93–6.
[30] Crameri R. Recombinant *Aspergillus fumigatus* allergens: from the nucleotide sequences to clinical applications. Int Arch Allergy Immunol 1998;115:99–114.
[31] Chapman MD, Smith AM, Vailes LD, et al. Recombinant allergens for diagnosis and therapy of allergic disease. J Allergy Clin Immunol 2000;106(3):409–18.
[32] Crameri R. High throughput screening: a rapid way to recombinant allergens. Allergy 2001; 56(Suppl 67):30–4.
[33] Valenta R, Kraft D. From allergen structure to new forms of allergen-specific immunotherapy. Curr Opin Immunol 2002;14(4):718–27.
[34] Wallner M, Gruber P, Radauer C, et al. La scale and medium scale production of recombinant allergens in *Escherichia coli*. Methods 2004;32(3):219–26.

[35] Dudler T, Chen WQ, Wang S, et al. High-level expression in *Escherichia coli* and rapid purification of enzymatically active honey bee venom phospholipase A_2. Biochim Biophys Acta 1992;1165(2):201–10.
[36] Müller UR, Dudler T, Schneider T, et al. Type I skin reactivity to native and recombinant phospholipase A_2 from honey bee venom is similar. J Allergy Clin Immunol 1995;96(3): 395–402.
[37] Forster E, Dudler T, Gmachl M, et al. Natural and recombinant enzymatically active or inactive bee venom phospholipase A_2 has the same potency to release histamine from basophils in patients with Hymenoptera allergy. J Allergy Clin Immunol 1995;95(6):1229–35.
[38] Schneider T, Lang AB, Carballido JM, et al. Human monoclonal or polyclonal antibodies recognize predominantly discontinuous epitopes on bee venom phospholipase PLA_2. J Allergy Clin Immunol 1994;94(1):61–70.
[39] Wymann D, Akdis CA, Blesken T, et al. Enzymatic activity of soluble phospholipase PLA_2 does not affect the specific IgE, IgG4 and cytokine responses in bee sting allergy. Clin Exp Allergy 1998;29(7):839–49.
[40] Müller U, Fricker M, Wymann D, et al. Increased specificity of diagnostic tests with recombinant major bee venom allergen phospholipase A_2. Clin Exp Allergy 1997;27(8):915–20.
[41] Hoffmann-Sommergruber K, O′Riordain G, Ahorn H, et al. Molecular characterization of Dau c 1, the Bet v 1 homologous protein from carrot and its cross-reactivity with Bet v 1 and Api g 1. Clin Exp Allergy 1999;29(6):840–7.
[42] Tresch S, Holzmann D, Baumann S, et al. *In vitro* and *in vivo* allergenicity of recombinant Bet v 1 compared to the reactivity of natural birch pollen extract. Clin Exp Allergy 2003;33(8): 1153–8.
[43] Schmid-Grendelmeier P, Crameri R. Recombinant allergens for skin testing. Int Arch Allergy Immunol 2001;125(2):96–111.
[44] Schmid-Grendelmeier P, Holzmann D, Himly M, et al. Native Art v 1 and recombinant Art v 1 are able to induce humoral and T cell-mediated *in vitro* and *in vivo* responses in mugwort allergy. J Allergy Clin Immunol 2003;111(6):1328–36.
[45] Crameri R, Lidholm J, Grönlund H, et al. Automated specific IgE assay with recombinant allergens: evaluation of the recombinant *Aspergillus fumigatus* allergen I in the Pharmacia CAP System. Clin Exp Allergy 1996;26(12):1411–9.
[46] Hiller R, Laffer S, Harwanegg C, et al. Microarrayed allergen molecules: diagnostic gatekeepers for allergy treatment. FASEB J 2002;16:414–6.
[47] Allergome: a platform for allergen knowledge. Available at: www.allergome.org. Accessed December 28, 2006.
[48] Heiss S, Mahler V, Steiner R, et al. Component-resolved diagnosis (CRD) of type I allergy with recombinant grass and tree pollen allergens by skin testing. J Invest Dermatol 1999; 113(5):830–7.
[49] Valenta R, Lidholm J, Niederberger V, et al. The recombinant allergen-based concept of component-resolved diagnostics and immunotherapy (CRD and CRIT). Clin Exp Allergy 1999;29(7):896–904.
[50] Aalberse RC, van der Gaag R, van Leeuwen J. Serologic aspects of IgG4 antibodies. J Immunol 1983;130:722–6.
[51] Akdis CA, Blesken T, Wymann D, et al. Differential regulation of human T cell cytokine patterns and IgE and IgG4 responses by conformational antigen variants. Eur J Immunol 1998; 28(3):914–25.
[52] Carballido JM, Carballido-Perrig N, Kägi MK, et al. T cell epitope specificity in human allergic and non-allergic individuals to bee venom phospholipase A_2. J Immunol 1993;91: 3582–91.
[53] Dudler T, Altmann F, Carballido JM, et al. Carbohydrate-dependent, HLA class II-restricted, human T cell response to the bee venom allergen phospholipase A_2 in allergic patients. Eur J Immunol 1995;25:538–42.

[54] Blaser K, Carballido JM, Faith A, et al. Determinants and mechanisms of human immune responses to bee venom phospholipase A_2. Int Arch Allergy Immunol 1998;117:1–10.
[55] Müller U, Akdis CA, Fricker M, et al. Successful immunotherapy with T-cell epitope peptides of bee venom phospholipase A_2 induces specific T-cell anergy in patients allergic to bee venom. J Allergy Clin Immunol 1998;101:747–54.
[56] Flückiger S, Limacher A, Glaser AG, et al. Structural aspects of cross-reactive allergens. Recent Research Developments in Allergy and Clinical Immunology 2004;5:57–75.
[57] Stadler MB, Stadler BM. Allergenicity prediction by protein sequence. FASEB J 2003;17: 1141–3.
[58] Li KB, Issac P, Krishnan A. Predicting allergenic proteins using wavlet transform. Bioinformatics 2004;20:2572–8.
[59] Valenta R, Duchene M, Ebner C, et al. Profilins constitute a novel family of functional plant pan-allergens. J Exp Med 1992;175:377–85.
[60] Reese G, Ayuso R, Lehrer SB. Tropomyosin: an invertebrate pan-allergen. Int Arch Allergy Immunol 1999;119:247–58.
[61] Barral P, Batanero E, Palomares O, et al. A major allergen from pollen defines a novel family of plant proteins and shows intra- and interspecies cross-reactivity. J Immunol 2004;172: 3644–51.
[62] Flückiger S, Fijten H, Whitley P, et al. Cyclophilins, a new family of cross-reactive allergens. Eur J Immunol 2002;32:10–7.
[63] Limacher A, Glaser AG, Meier C, et al. Cross-reactivity and 1.4 Å crystal structure of *Malassezia sympodialis* Thioredoxin (Mala s 13), a member of a new pan-allergen family. J Immunol 2007;178:389–96.
[64] Ferreira F, Hirtenlehner K, Jelek A, et al. Dissection of immunoglobulin E and T lymphocyte reactivity of isoforms of the major birch pollen allergen Bet v 1: potential use of hypoallergenic isoforms for immunotherapy. J Exp Med 1996;183:599–609.
[65] Valenta R, Sperr WR, Ferreira F, et al. Induction of specific histamine release from basophils with purified natural and recombinant birch pollen allergens. J Allergy Clin Immunol 1993; 91:88–97.
[66] Linhart B, Valenta R. Molecular design of allergy vaccines. Curr Opin Immunol 2005;17: 646–55.
[67] Hoffmann-Sommergruber K, Demoly P, Crameri R, et al. IgE reactivity to Api g 1, a major celery allergen, in a Central European population is based on primary sensitization to Bet v 1. J Allergy Clin Immunol 1999;104:478–84.
[68] May Y, Gadermaier G, Bohle B, et al. Mutational analysis of amino acid positions crucial for IgE-binding epitopes of the major apple (*Malus domestica*) allergen, Mal d 1. Int Arch Allergy Immunol 2006;139:53–62.
[69] Bohle B, Radakovics A, Luttkopf D, et al. Characterization of the T cell response to the major hazelnut allergen, Cor a 1.04: evidence for a relevant T cell epitope not cross-reactive with homologous pollen allergens. Clin Exp Allergy 2005;35:1392–9.
[70] Reuter A, Fortunato D, Garoffo LP, et al. Novel isoforms of Pru av 1 with diverging immunoglobulin E binding properties identified by a synergistic combination of molecular biology and proteomics. Proteomics 2005;5:282–9.
[71] Breiteneder H, Ebner C. Molecular and biochemical classification of plant-derived food allergens. J Allergy Clin Immunol 2000;1067:27–36.
[72] Wagner S, Sowka S, Mayer C, et al. Identification of a *Heave brasiliensis* latex manganese superoxide dismutase (Hev b 10) as a cross-reactive allergen. Int Arch Allergy Immunol 2001;125:120–7.
[73] Andersson A, Rasool O, Schmidt M, et al. Cloning, expression and characterization of two new IgE-binding proteins from the yeast *Malassezia sympodialis* with sequence similarities to heat shock proteins and manganese superoxide dismutase. Eur J Biochem 2004;271: 1885–94.

[74] Radauer C, Willerroider M, Fuchs H, et al. Cross-reactive and species-specific immunoglobulin E epitopes of plant profilins: an experimental and structure-based analysis. Clin Exp Allergy 2006;36:920–9.

[75] Mellon MB, Frank BT, Fang KC. Mast cell alpha-chymase reduces IgE recognition of birch pollen profilin by cleaving antibody-binding epitopes. J Immunol 2002;168:290–7.

[76] Das Dores S, Chopin C, Romano A, et al. IgE-binding and cross-reactivity of a new 41 kDa allergen of codfish. Allergy 2002;57(Suppl 72):84–7.

[77] Bernard H, Negroni L, Chatel JM, et al. Molecular basis of IgE cross-reactivity between human beta-casein and bovine beta-casein, a major allergen of milk. Mol Immunol 2000;37: 161–7.

[78] Maynard F, Chatel JM, Wal JM. Immunological IgE cross-reactions of bovine and human alpha-lactalbumins in cow's milk allergic patients. Food and Agricultural Immunology 1999;11:179–89.

[79] Baur X, Bossert J, Koops F. IgE-mediated allergy to recombinant human insulin in a diabetic. Allergy 2003;58:676–8.

[80] Pandjaitan B, Swoboda I, Brandejsky-Pichler F, et al. *Escherichia coli* expression and purification of recombinant dog albumin, a cross-reactive animal allergen. J Allergy Clin Immunol 2000;105:279–85.

[81] Natter S, Seibeler S, Hufnagl P, et al. Isolation of cDNA clones coding for IgE autoantigens with serum IgE from atopic dermatitis patients. FASEB J 1998;12:1559–69.

[82] Crameri R, Kodzius R, Konthur Z, et al. Tapping allergen repertoires by advanced cloning technologies. Int Arch Allergy Immunol 2001;124:43–7.

[83] Appenzeller U, Meyer C, Menz G, et al. IgE-mediated reactions to autoantigens in allergic diseases. Int Arch Allergy Immunol 1999;118:193–6.

[84] Mayer C, Hemmann S, Faith A, et al. Cloning, production, characterization and IgE cross-reactivity of different manganese superoxide dismutases in individuals sensitized to *Aspergillus fumigatus*. Int Arch Allergy Immunol 1997;113:213–5.

[85] Crameri R, Faith A, Hemmann S, et al. Humoral and cell-mediated autoimmunity in allergy to *Aspergillus fumigatus*. J Exp Med 1996;184:265–70.

[86] Flückiger S, Scapozza L, Mayer C, et al. Immunological and structural analysis of IgE-mediated cross-reactivity between manganese superoxide dismutases. Int Arch Allergy Immunol 2002;128:292–303.

[87] Flückiger S, Mittl PRE, Scapozza L, et al. Comparison of the crystal structures of the human manganese superoxide dismutase and the homologous *Aspergillus fumigatus* allergen at 2 Å resolution. J Immunol 2002;168:1267–72.

[88] Schmid-Grendelmeier P, Flückiger S, Disch R, et al. IgE-mediated and T cell-mediated autoimmunity against manganese superoxide dismutase in atopic dermatitis. J Allergy Clin Immunol 2005;115:1068–75.

[89] Schmid-Grendelmeier P, Scheynius A, Crameri R. The role of sensitization to *Malassezia sympodialis* in atopic eczema. Chem Immunol Allergy 2006;91:98–109.

[90] Mayer C, Appenzeller U, Seelbach H, et al. Humoral and cell-mediated autoimmune reactions to human acidic ribosomal P_2 protein in individuals sensitized to *Aspergillus fumigatus* P_2 protein. J Exp Med 1999;189:1507–12.

[91] Limacher A, Kloer DP, Flückiger S, et al. The crystal structure of *Aspergillus fumigatus* cyclophilin reveals 3D domain swapping of a central element. Structure 2006;14: 185–95.

[92] Glaser AG, Limacher A, Flückiger S, et al. Analysis of the cross-reactivity and of the 1.5 Å crystal structure of the *Malassezia sympodialis* Mala s 6 allergen, a member of the cyclophilin pan-allergen family. Biochem J 2006;396:41–9.

[93] Weichel M, Vergoossen NJ, Bonomi S, et al. Screening the allergenic repertoires of wheat and maize with sera from double-blind, placebo-controlled food challenge positive patients. Allergy 2006;61:128–35.

[94] Weichel M, Glaser AG, Ballmer-Weber BK, et al. Wheat and maize thioredoxins: a novel cross-reactive cereal allergen family related to baker's asthma. J Allergy Clin Immunol 2006;117:676–81.

[95] Neudecker P, Lehmann K, Nerkamp J, et al. Mutational epitope analysis of Pru av 1 and Api g 1, the major allergens of cherry (*Prunus avium*) celery (*Apium graveolens*): correlating IgE reactivity with three-dimensional structure. Biochem J 2003;376:97–107.

[96] Crameri R. Correlating IgE reactivity with three-dimensional structure. Biochem J 2003;276: e1–2.

[97] Valenta R, Seiberler S, Natter S, et al. Autoallergy: a pathogenetic factor in atopic dermatitis? J Allergy Clin Immunol 2000;105:432–7.

[98] Aalberse RC. Structural biology of allergens. J Allergy Clin Immunol 2000;106:228–38.

ELSEVIER
SAUNDERS

Immunol Allergy Clin N Am
27 (2007) 79–92

IMMUNOLOGY
AND ALLERGY
CLINICS
OF NORTH AMERICA

Recognition of Lipids from Pollens by CD1-Restricted T Cells

Fabrizio Spinozzi, MD[a,*], Steven A. Porcelli, MD[b,c]

[a] *Experimental Immunology and Allergy, Department of Clinical and Experimental Medicine, University of Perugia, Policlinico Monteluce, Via Brunamonti 51, I-06122 Perugia, Italy*
[b] *Department of Microbiology and Immunology, Albert Einstein College of Medicine, Room 416, Forchheimer Building, 1300 Morris Park Avenue, Bronx, NY 10461, USA*
[c] *Department of Internal Medicine, Albert Einstein College of Medicine, Room 416, Forchheimer Building, 1300 Morris Park Avenue, Bronx, NY 10461, USA*

Phospholipids (PLs) and glycolipids account for more than 50% of membrane structures of pollen grains. These lipids are an integral component of pollen grain structure, and play a dynamic role in transport of the pollen grain contents across membranes; they are thus essential for the relevant physiologic role of pollens in sexual reproduction in higher plants [1]. Although the importance of the lipid constituents of pollens has been widely appreciated by plant biologists from many years, the potential importance of pollen lipids to allergic responses has been largely ignored by immunologists who have focused exclusively on the immunogenic properties of protein constituents of the pollen grains and their relevance to allergy in susceptible individuals. In recently published and ongoing studies, the authors have investigated the importance of the lipid constituents of pollen grains to the immune responses that can occur to these important environmental allergens. Building on new advances in the study of lipid antigen presentation to T cells by the CD1 family of antigen-presenting molecules, they have found intriguing new evidence pointing to a potentially important role for pollen lipids in the stimulation of allergic responses.

This work was supported by grants from the University of Perugia, Italy (PROGAT.DELFA99) to F.S., and the National Insititutes of Health, USA (AI45889), and the Hirschl Trust to S.A.P.

* Corresponding author.
E-mail address: spinozzi@unipg.it (F. Spinozzi).

doi:10.1016/j.iac.2006.11.004 ***immunology.theclinics.com***

CD1 molecules and the presentation of lipid antigens to T cells

CD1 molecules are β2-microglobulin associated surface glycoproteins that bear significant structural similarity to MHC class I molecules [2]. In humans, the CD1 family consists of five members, designated CD1a, CD1b, CD1c, CD1d, and CD1e. Based on homology relationships and the details of their expression and function, CD1a, -b, -c, and -e are classified as group 1 CD1 molecules. CD1d composes a separate group, and is the only member of the group 2 CD1 molecules [3]. Both group 1 and group 2 CD1 molecules are lipid-binding proteins that are expressed on specialized antigen-presenting cells (APC), including myeloid dendritic cells (DCs), on which they perform the role of presenting foreign and self-lipids and glycolipids to T cells. In marked contrast to the highly polymorphic MHC-encoded protein antigen-presenting molecules, CD1 proteins show extremely limited polymorphism between individuals of a given species [4]. The group 1 CD1 molecules have been characterized most extensively in humans and have been demonstrated to present microbial lipid antigens and certain self-lipids to a diverse group of T cells [5]. Group 2 CD1 molecules (ie, CD1d) have been more deeply studied in humans and also in a wide variety of experimental mouse models, which is made possible because CD1d is the only member of the CD1 family that is conserved in rodents. CD1d has been identified in mice and humans as the critical antigen-presenting molecule that controls the development and function of an unusual population of regulatory T cells known as invariant natural killer T (iNKT) cells (Vα24i NKT cells in humans and Vα14i NKT cells in mice) [3,5]. This ability to use mouse models for analysis of CD1d has greatly facilitated the study of its role in a wide variety of disease processes, including models of protein antigen–induced allergic airway disease [6]. Our recent work extends the involvement of CD1 to human allergic airway diseases, and suggests an important role for the CD1 system in presentation of pollen-derived lipids in common allergic diseases associated with seasonal exposure to specific plant pollens.

The importance of lipids in pollen grain structure and function

Pollen grains, which contain sperm cells complete with plasma membranes, are structurally characterized by a unique pollen wall that is generally subdivided into three principal strata: (1) an outer exine composed of the chemically resistant polymer sporopollenin; (2) an inner intine made primarily of cellulose; and (3) a pollen coat, composed of lipids, proteins, pigments, and aromatic compounds, that fills the sculptured cavities of the outer exine [7]. The exine principal constituent sporopollenin is not a unique substance but rather a series of related biopolymers derived from largely saturated precursors, such as fatty acids [8]. Moreover, there is now extensive evidence that the proteins and lipids in the pollen coat contribute to stigma adhesion, thus realizing the first contact necessary for plant reproduction.

The subsequent hydration of compatible grains leads to the activation of pollen metabolism. Disrupting pollen coat lipids or pollen coat proteins in *Brassicaceae* species can delay or block pollen hydration resulting in male sterility [9].

With the principal objective of studying the relationships of the lipid constituents of pollen grains to the immune responses of allergic subjects, we analyzed in detail the lipids contained in pollens from European cypress trees that are known to strongly evoke seasonal allergic symptoms in susceptible subjects. Analyzing the lipid composition of the membranes from *Cupressus arizonica* and *C. sempervirens* by two-dimensional thin layer chromatography (TLC), we were able to recognize a variety of PLs that are similar to those previously described for *Typha latifolia* or *Brassica napus* pollens [10,11]. PL content in 1 mg of cypress pollen grains is about 10 nmol, corresponding to 60.3%. Phosphatidyl choline (PC) represents greater than 50% of total PLs, followed by phosphatidyl ethanolamine (PE; 15%) and then smaller amounts of the other PL classes, such as phosphatidyl serine (PS) and phosphatidic acid. Molecular species compositions of TLC-purified pollen PC and PE determined by tandem MS/MS exhibit a restricted distribution dominated by species containing the fatty acid linoleate ($C18{:}2_{n\text{-}6}$), such that the major species in each case are dioleoyl (18:2/18:2). There are no disaturated or monounsaturated species in either PC or PE from cypress pollen grains. Conversely, glycolipids represent 39.7% of total pollen lipids, corresponding to 6.6 nmol/mg.

Possible relevance of external lipids in pollen grain capture

The respiratory tract contains several cell types, including epithelial cells, macrophages, and DCs capable of interacting with inhaled pollens to function as APC. The mechanisms of recognition of pollen grains as allergens by the immune system have been debated for a considerable time, with diverse views depending on the biochemical substances considered as the principal true allergens and their localization within the pollen grain [12]. Because most of the proteins described as sensitizing agents are contained inside the intine membrane or in the cytoplasmic region [13], it is difficult to explain their rapid delivery in vivo to the host immune system. Traditional models suggest that nonspecific receptors, such as C-type lectins and integrins, rapidly bind surface glycoproteins, favoring phagocytosis by alveolar macrophages of the whole pollen grain or of starch granules (<5 μm) derived from grasses [14]. Subsequent direct interaction of T-cell receptor (TCR) with antigen-derived peptides presented by MHC-encoded antigen-presenting molecules [15] defines a current central paradigm in immunology. Both upper [16] and lower airways [17] are known to contain large numbers of DCs often expressing high levels of CD1a protein [18], particularly in asthmatics as compared with other pulmonary diseases [19]. Recently we have studied the expression of CD1d proteins, and the previously described CD1a, at the surface of DCs to evaluate the hypothesis that these CD1 proteins may act as cell surface receptors that capture pollens within the respiratory tract. As outlined earlier, such a hypothesis is justified by the demonstration that species-specific pollen-stigma adhesion is mediated by hydrophobic (lipid) molecules in the pollen exine and external coat [1,7–11].

To this end we chose for study the cypress allergy model, which is unique because patients are often monosensitive with seasonal respiratory symptoms occurring exclusively in winter months, from January to March [20]. Moreover, the cypress pollen grains are inaperturate (ie, lack pores in the pollen wall), do not contain starch granules, but demonstrate protuberances in the outer exine membrane consistent with those described as hexagonal phase structures in liposome membranes [21]. We observed in samples derived from bronchoalveolar lavage fluid of asthmatics that pulmonary macrophages and DCs capture the whole pollen grain. This observation was associated with a concomitant increase in frequency of CD1d^{+} DCs, which was not seen in control samples (Fig. 1). Dendritic cells can be derived from circulating monocytes cultured with IL-4 and GM-CSF and used as antigen-presenting cells (see Fig. 1). Following CD1-dependent binding to the DC surface, the subsequent ingestion of the whole pollen material was evident starting at 15 minutes and leading to a progressive concentration over the time of pollen-derived material within endoplasmic organelles [22]. A possible explanation for this finding is that non-bilayer PL arrangements (hexagonally packed cylinders of the hexagonal tubular phase) occur in about 40% of membrane lipids from pollens, particularly phosphatidyl-serine, cardiolipin, PE, and PC. Electron microscopy studies demonstrate that these non-bilayer structures appear as protuberances on the surface of the membrane [23]. In this manner, acyl side chains of PLs are exposed and may enter the CD1 pocket, making the contact between pollen grain and dendritic cell stable. DCs thus have the capacity to bind surface pollen lipids by specific interaction with CD1 molecules, a fundamental step in tree pollen capture and phagocytosis by specialized antigen presenting cells.

CD1-restricted lipid-specific T cells in allergic diseases

Until now there has been no clear evidence that natural lipids from nonbacterial or nonmammalian species may be recognized as antigens in a CD1-restricted fashion by the human immune system, apart from the well-described responses of CD1d-restricted NKT cells to the glycolipid α-galactosyl ceramide extracted from marine sponges [24]. Vα14i NKT cells in mice have been described, however, that recognize natural and synthetic glycolipid and PL antigens in a CD1d-restricted manner [25], and recently this T-cell subset has been implicated in the development of allergen-induced airway hyperreactivity (AHR) in animal models and in human subjects [26].

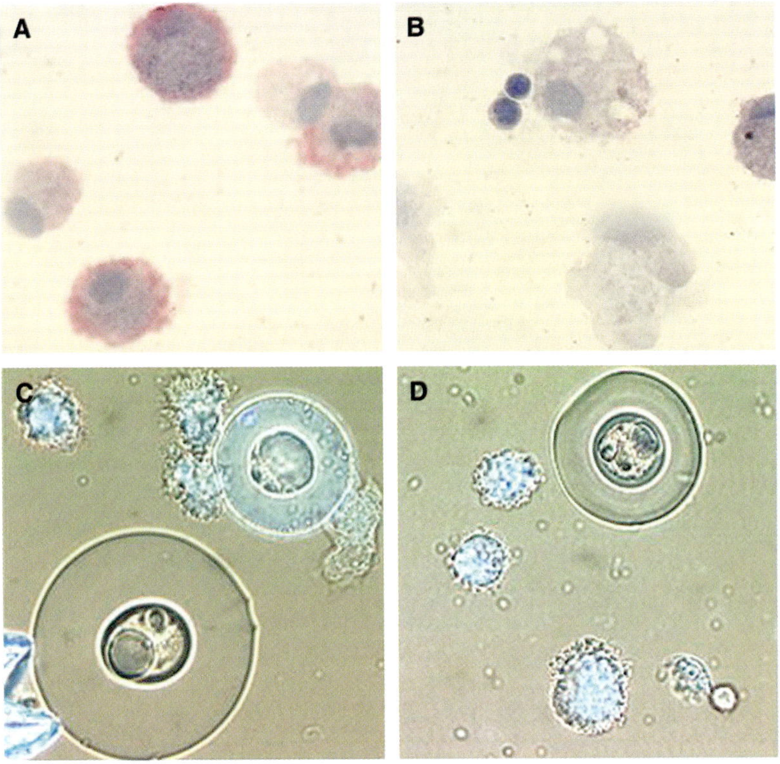

Fig. 1. Interactions between CD1d^{+} DCs and cypress pollen. (*A*) A bronchoalveolar lavage cytospin sample from asthmatic subject as it appeared after labelling with anti-human CD1d mAb and staining with alkaline phosphatase/antialkaline phosphatase technique. Cells with morphology consistent with macrophages and DCs show surface or intracellular staining. (*B*) Normal control sample does not displaye surface or cellular staining. (*C*) CD1d^{+} DCs can bind cypress pollen grains in vitro. (*D*) Pretreatment with a monoclonal antibody directed toward human CD1d completely blocked the binding of pollen grain.

In our studies we have had the opportunity to obtain blood samples and, in some cases, nasal mucosa specimens from cypress-sensitive subjects [22,27]. Because cypress pollination in Italy is a seasonal phenomenon typically present from January to March, we undertook a survey of the frequency of PL-specific T-cell lines in a subset of monosensitive subjects sampled at regular intervals over a 1-year period. Our initial studies used a semiquantitative approach to enumerate PL-specific T-cells in patients who had documented cypress pollen allergy and in normal controls. We found that the average numbers of PL-specific T-cell lines recovered from circulating mononuclear cells of allergic subjects after in vitro culture paralleled the presence of cypress pollen grains in the atmosphere (Fig. 2). Relatively high numbers were recovered during the pollinating period (ie, January to March), following the characteristic seasonal distribution. In

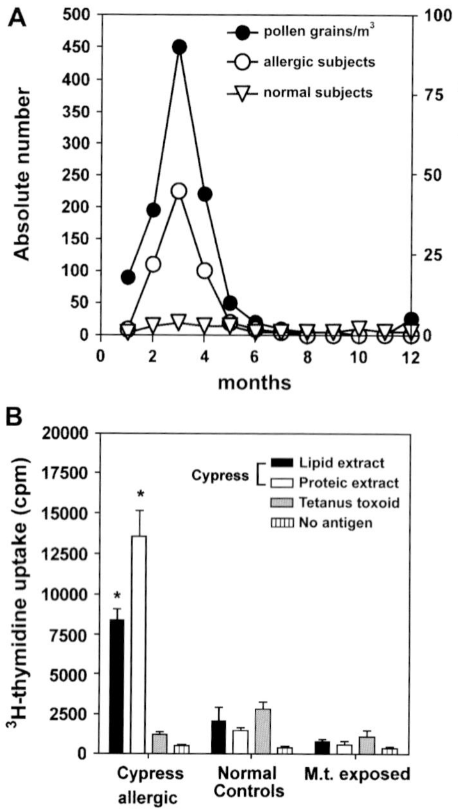

Fig. 2. Response to cypress pollen PLs in allergic subjects. (*A*) Correlation over 1-year period between atmospheric levels of cypress pollen in the region inhabited by the study subjects (as reported by National Aerobiological Society annual survey, www.isao.bo.cnr.it/aerobio/polline.html) and the frequency of PL-specific T-cell lines derived from the blood of the subjects. (*B*) Mean values (±SD) of proliferative responses of PBMC from cypress-sensitive subjects, normal controls, or *Mycobacterium*-exposed health care workers to stimulation with cypress antigens. Cypress-sensitive subjects displayed a clear response ($P < .005$) to PL and protein extracts from pollen compared with normal controls or *M. tuberculosis*–exposed subjects. (*From* Agea R, Russano A, Bistoni O, et al. Human CD-1 restricted recognition of lipids from proteins. J Exp Med 2005;202:295–308; with permission. Copyright © 2005, The Rockefeller University Press.)

contrast, there was no evidence of inducible PL-specific T-cell lines in the peripheral blood of allergic subjects sampled during nonpollinating periods (from May to December). Moreover, a clear response to pollen lipid extract was seen in allergic subjects, as compared with normal controls or *Mycobacterium tuberculosis*–exposed subjects (see Fig. 2) In particular, PC, phosphatidyl-glycerol (PG), and PE were determined to be the major antigenic substances able to induce the seasonal expansion of group 1 and group 2 CD1-restricted T cells, most of which appeared to be similar to classic

$CD4^+$ T cells expressing αβ TCRs, although occasional examples of PL-reactive Vα24i NKT cells and γδ TCR^+ T cells were also isolated from allergic subjects. T-cell clones derived from most of the PL-reactive lines secreted Th1- and Th2-type cytokines, and many of these possessed functional properties characteristic of regulatory T cells (ie, IL-10 and TGF-β production). Some of these T cells displayed strong reactivity toward unsaturated (16:0 or 18:0) PLs. Unsaturated PLs are virtually absent in the pollen grain, but are known constituents of mammalian tissues, such as pulmonary surfactant and brain tissue in humans. The PL composition of human respiratory surfactant [28] is frequently altered during allergic respiratory diseases [29]. We thus speculate that cross-reactivity between CD1-restricted T cells primed by pollen-derived PLs with similar self-PLs containing C16:0 or C18:0 acyl chains may explain the self-perpetuation of the immune response to pollen-derived allergens frequently seen even outside the pollinating season [30]. Consistent with this possibility is the observation that humans who had mild asthma who received a natural porcine surfactant preparation consisting of 99% PLs had unexpectedly worsened pulmonary inflammation following allergen challenge [31].

Despite the presence of increased numbers of $CD1^+$ DCs in the airways of asthmatics, no definitive proof currently exists that lipid-specific CD1-restricted T cells can effectively lead to clinically defined allergic diseases. Animal models suggest that Vα14i NKT cells are fundamental for the stimulation of AHR in the ovalbumin-induced mouse model of allergic asthma [6,26]. Mice lacking these CD1d-restricted T cells, because of gene knockouts in either *TCRAJ18* locus (required for the invariant TCRα chain expressed by these T cells) or the *CD1D* locus (required for thymic positive selection of developing iNKT cells), show markedly reduced airway inflammation and asthma following challenge with the sensitizing protein antigen [6,32,33]. Based on adoptive transfer experiments, it seems that the production of IL-4 and IL-13 by iNKT cells is at least one component of their essential role in promoting AHR [6]. An important and as yet unresolved aspect of this model is the question of what specific antigens or other stimuli are driving the cytokine production by iNKT cells in the lungs of sensitized animals. It is extremely unlikely that these CD1-restricted, lipid-reactive iNKT cells are responding directly to the OVA protein used for the challenge. A more likely hypothesis is that they are activated by recognition of endogenous lipid ligands that may be exposed by the inflammatory milieu in the lung, or by ubiquitous environmental or microbial lipid ligands that find their way into the bronchial tree.

Recent studies also show that the iNKT activator KRN7000, a synthetic glycolipid in the α-galactosylceramide (αGalCer) family, has a major effect on modulating the development of AHR when given to mice before challenge in the OVA hypersensitivity model [34]. Systemic or intranasal KRN7000 administration shortly before airway challenge with OVA in sensitized mice inhibits elicitation of AHR. This effect may be considered in some ways paradoxical, given that KRN7000 is a strong activator of iNKT cells and these cells clearly are capable of making copious amounts of cytokines, such as IL-4, IL-5, and IL-13, that are associated with worsening or induction of AHR. Several possible mechanisms for this effect are under consideration, including the potential for KRN7000 to induce a dominant Th1-type response that negates the effects of the Th2 cytokines that are produced or the documented ability of KRN7000 to induce a state of iNKT cell anergy or depletion under some conditions [35]. Although the mechanism for the striking ability of KRN7000 to inhibit AHR in this model is not yet clearly understood, this finding strongly suggests a therapeutic approach to rhinitis and asthma in humans through the administration of lipid-based agonists or antagonists of iNKT cells. This possibility is made even more intriguing by recent reports of an extraordinarily high frequency of iNKT cells localizing to the airways of humans who have allergic asthma [36,37]. There is a debate concerning the real frequency of iNKT cells in the BAL fluid of asthmatic children and adults who have mild to moderate disease, however [36,38], and also in our experience the frequency of $CD4^+$ $V\alpha24i$ NKT cells usually does not exceed 10% of total $CD4^+$ lymphocytes in the BAL fluid of asthmatic subjects (F. Spinozzi and colleagues, unpublished observations, 2006). Although it remains plausible that CD1d-restricted $V\alpha24i$ NKT cells play a significant role in allergic airway inflammation, it should be kept in mind that other lipid-specific T cells exist at mucosal surfaces and that these may have equal or even greater importance. Notably, these could include classic $CD4^+$ $TCR\alpha\beta^+$ T cells, or $TCR\gamma\delta^+$ T cells that are either $CD4^+$ or double-negative (ie, lacking CD4 and CD8 expression), which our studies suggest have the capacity to drive a lipid antigen-specific inflammatory response in cypress pollen–sensitive subjects [22,25,27]. Additional work is needed to achieve a complete pathologic picture and this should include characterization of fine antigen specificity of resident mucosal T-cell clones using natural, well-characterized phospho- and glycolipids from pollens and an extensive panel of related synthetic lipid antigens. In this way, insight could be gained into the question of which T-cell populations among those described as having the capacity to respond to lipid antigen stimulation at the mucosal surfaces are most likely to be the predominant ones responsible for triggering or perpetuating AHR and other allergic reactions.

Mucosal $\gamma\delta$ T cells and lipid antigens

The authors were among the first to consider unconventional T lymphocytes at the sites of mucosal inflammation as key regulatory cells for the development of asthma [39]. It has been proposed that $\gamma\delta$ T cells complement $\alpha\beta$ T cells by providing a rapidly induced, but weaker, response before the $\alpha\beta$ T-cell activation has fully developed. This suggestion is based on the cytokine secretion pattern of $\gamma\delta$ T cells and their ability to be restricted by nonclassic MHC-like molecules, such as CD1 [40]. To this purpose, animal studies have yielded conflicting results in recent years. Initially, γδ T cells, which represent a consistent resident cellular subset in the respiratory tract of mice [41], were believed to act as suppressive regulatory cells in IgE-mediated allergic responses [42]. Human $CD4^{+}\gamma\delta^{+}$ T cells activated in vitro have been shown to provide a contact signal that can induce B cells to switch to IgE production in the presence of IL-4 [43], and expansion of γδ T cells in the human nasal mucosa of allergic subjects has been described [44]. Our own studies have stressed the expansion of an oligoclonal $CD4^{+}$ γδ T-cell subset bearing Vδ1 TCRs in the airways of untreated allergic asthmatic patients [45]. These cells, virtually absent in the airways of normal subjects, were able to respond in vitro to the specific allergen and to produce IL-4, a finding that prompted us to define them as allergen-specific T cells [46].

By studying subjects who have seasonal allergic rhinitis to cypress pollen, we have obtained from nasal turbinates several γδ T-cell clones that respond specifically to pollen-derived PL antigens. These clones are $V\delta1^{+}$ and $CD4^{+}$, and half of them coexpress the CD161 molecule, thus confirming the expansion of mucosal $V\delta1^{+}CD4^{+}$ T lymphocytes described in subjects suffering from rhinitis [44] or asthma [45]. PE is the main PL to which these γδ T-cell clones respond in vitro, and their recognition of PE is CD1d-restricted. Blocking experiments with mAbs against CD1 epitopes showed that PE reactivity depended largely on CD1d molecules expressed by APCs. Assays of IL-2 production by mucosal-derived γδ T-cell clones from allergic subjects in vitro revealed that unsaturated 16:0/18:2 PE together with 18:2/18:2 PE were the main compounds to which such clones responded. Saturated PE species and other natural PLs from animal sources, such as brain and chicken egg PE, and 16:0/16:0 PC were not stimulatory.

Current knowledge about lipid antigen recognition by γδ T-cell clones has been extremely limited, although previous studies have shown the potential for self-reactivity of $V\delta1^{+}$ T cells that is restricted by CD1c [40]. These T cells are usually double-negative, do not express the CD161 receptor (NKR-P1A), and produce almost exclusively IFN-γ. The candidate self-lipid antigens they recognize are not known, but it is speculated that they may be mannosyl-1-phosphodolichols that are structurally related to the mycobacterial hexosyl-1-phosphoisoprenoids presented by CD1c to αβ T cells [47]. Our recent evidence that mucosal γδ T cells from subjects with rhinitis can recognize PLs from pollens, together with the fact that the rapid mucosal capture of pollen grains by APCs can be mediated by CD1 molecules, could lead to the conclusion that lipid-specific CD1d-restricted γδ T cells may function as first-line responders in the mucosa. In this role, these enigmatic T cells could prove to be key regulators of cytokines, chemokines, and other factors determining the inflammatory environment that governs the onset and persistence of allergic responses.

Th2 properties of lipid-specific CD1-restricted T cells

The main functional characteristics of allergen-specific T cells are the capacity to help autologous B cells in IgE production and the secretion of the so-called "Th2-type cytokines" (IL-4, IL-5, and IL-13), which induce many of the characteristic features of airway inflammation [48]. That some T cells in allergic subjects may recognize lipid from pollens in a CD1-restricted fashion does not necessarily mean that these are functionally relevant to induction of allergic responses. There is a growing body of evidence, however, that CD1-restricted lipid-reactive T cells are capable of producing a wide array of cytokines, including those that are characteristic of classic Th2 lymphocytes [5,6,49]. Considerable functional and phenotypic heterogeneity has been shown for lipid-antigen–specific T cell clones, and in some cases individual clones capable of secreting Th1- and Th2-type cytokines (ie, Th0 cells) have been described [5]. In addition, some clones have been found under appropriate conditions of lipid stimulation to secrete relevant amounts of highly immunosuppressive cytokines, such as IL-10 and transforming growth factor β (TGFβ). In our preliminary observations we have noted that some PL-reactive $V\alpha24i^{+}$ NKT cells, and some TCR $\gamma\delta^{+}$ T-cell clones, displayed a cytokine production pattern similar to that of regulatory T cells [50]. The in vitro responses of these T-cell clones are directed toward synthetic saturated PLs (C16:0) not usually present in pollen grain membranes. The polyclonal in vivo expansion of CD1-restricted lipid-reactive T lymphocytes at the mucosal surfaces of allergic subjects does not exclude the possibility that the recognition of self-PLs may trigger regulatory functions that could potentially attenuate allergic responses against exogenous PLs.

Another particular functional property we have observed in preliminary studies of CD1-restricted T-cell clones derived from allergic subjects is the ability to help autologous B cells to secrete IgE in vitro. Such a property, which is typical of classic Th2 T cells, is fundamentally linked to the ability to secrete large amounts of IL-4 and is likely to contribute to immunopathology in allergic responses. In our experience peripheral blood-derived TCR $\alpha\beta^{+}$ T-cell clones coexpressing the CD161 NKT cell marker were less efficient than their counterparts not expressing CD161 in favoring the IgE production in vitro. Moreover, $TCR\gamma\delta^{+}$ T-cell clones derived from nasal mucosa of allergic subjects were able to produce IL-4 and to induce IgE secretion by autologous non-T cells on PE stimulation. The capacity to help IgE production was present in $\gamma\delta^{+}CD4^{+}$ $CD161^{-}$ and $CD4^{+}CD161^{+}$ clones, whereas γδ T cell clones from normal subjects, even if able to secrete IL-4 in response to synthetic 16:0/18:2 PE or brain and egg PE, neither proliferated against pollen-derived PE nor produced IgE in vitro.

In parallel with the property of providing help for the production of IgE in vitro, we also investigated whether significant amounts of PL-specific IgE could be detected in the circulation of cypress pollen–allergic subjects

(Fig. 3). To this purpose, we initially analyzed the ability of natural or synthetic PLs to induce an immediate wheal and flare reaction when applied on the forearms of sensitive subjects. Natural (derived from cypress and olive pollens) and synthetic (C16:0/18:2 PC, PE, and PG; C18:2/18:2 PC and PE) PL suspensions gave appreciable reactions compared with those elicited by the vehicle substances or buffer alone. Moreover, olive-derived PE was less able than cypress-derived PE to trigger cutaneous hyperreactivity in cypress-sensitive subjects, but was able to bind to their circulating IgE. Because of the similarities in PL composition of pollens, olive-derived PE has also been able to induce some functional activation in PE-specific γδ T-cell clones derived from nasal mucosa of cypress-sensitive subjects. This finding is in line with the lack of polymorphism of CD1 receptors that might be the adaptive consequence of binding lipid antigens with conserved hydrophobic moieties [5].

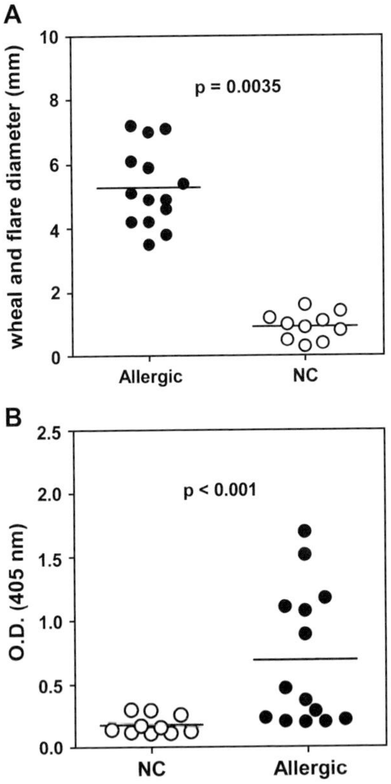

Fig. 3. IgE reactivity toward pollen PLs. (*A*) Average of mean wheal and flare reactions to cypress-derived PLs in allergic subjects and normal controls. (*B*) Circulating PE-specific IgE (mean optical densities at 405 nm) as detected by ELISA assay. (*From* Agea R, Russano A, Bistoni O, et al. Human CD-1 restricted recognition of lipids from proteins. J Exp Med 2005;202: 295–308; with permission. Copyright © 2005, The Rockefeller University Press.)

Summary

It is only recently that T-cell recognition of lipid antigens through the CD1-dependent pathway of presentation has been defined in detail. Now that this new mechanism for antigen-specific T cell activation is well established and moderately well understood, many studies are being initiated to evaluate its potential relevance to normal immune function and various disease states. In this regard, the studies reviewed in this article indicate a strong possibility that CD1-dependent presentation of exogenous lipids may be an important and previously unsuspected aspect of allergic diseases. Our studies focusing on T-cell responses to cypress pollen-derived PLs represent some of the first insights into this area, which could potentially extend to immune responses against a wide variety of plant-derived lipid antigens. This area of research thus has the potential to open up new concepts in the understanding of a range of allergic diseases and may also point to new approaches for diagnosis, therapy, and prevention.

References

[1] Mariani C, Wolters-Arts M. Complex waxes. Plant Cell 2000;12:1795–8.
[2] Moody DB, Zajonc DM, Wilson IA. Anatomy of CD1-lipid antigen complexes. Nat Rev Immunol 2005;5:387–99.
[3] Porcelli SA. The CD1 family. A third lineage of antigen-presenting molecules. Adv Immunol 1995;59:1–98.
[4] Han M, Hannick LI, DiBrino M, et al. Polymorphism of human CD1 genes. Tissue Antigens 1999;54:122–7.
[5] De Libero G, Mori L. Recognition of lipid antigens by T cells. Nat Rev Immunol 2005;5: 485–96.
[6] Akbari O, Stock P, Meyer E, et al. Essential role of NKT cells producing IL-4 and IL-13 in the development of allergen-induced airway hyperreactivity. Nat Med 2003;9:582–8.
[7] Edlund AF, Swanson R, Preuss D. Pollen and stigma structure and function: the role of diversity in pollination. Plant Cell 2004;16:S84–97.
[8] Giulford WJ, Schnider DM, Labovitz J, et al. High resolution solid state 13C-NMR spectroscopy of sporopollenins from different plant taxa. Plant Physiol 1988;86:134–6.
[9] Preuss D, Lemieux B, Yen G, et al. A conditional sterile mutation eliminate surface components from Arabidopsis pollen and disrupts cell signalling during fertilization. Genes Dev 1993;7:974–85.
[10] Caffrey M, Werner BG, Priestley DA. A crystalline lipid phase in a dry biological system: evidence from X-ray diffraction analysis of *Typha latifolia* pollen. Biochim Biophys Acta 1987;921:124–34.
[11] Hernandez-Pinzon I, Ross JH, Barnes KA, et al. Composition and role of tapetal lipid bodies in the biogenesis of the pollen coat of *Brassica napus*. Planta 1999;208:588–98.
[12] Driessen MN, Quanjer PH. Pollen deposition in intrathoracic airways. Eur Respir J 1991;4: 359–63.
[13] Grote M. In situ localization of pollen allergens by immunogold electron microscopy: allergens at unexpected sites. Int Arch Allergy Immunol 1999;118:1–6.
[14] Currie AJ, Stewart GA, McWilliam AS. Alveolar macrophages bind and phagocytose allergen-containing pollen starch granules via C-type lectin and integrin receptors: implications for airway inflammatory disease. J Immunol 2000;164:3878–86.

[15] Wilson IA, Garcia KC. T-cell receptor structure and TcR complexes. Curr Opin Struct Biol 1997;7:839–48.
[16] Fokkens VJ, Vinke JG, De Jong SS, et al. Differences in the cellular infiltrate in the adenoid of allergic children compared with age- and gender-matched controls. Clin Exp Allergy 1998; 28:187–95.
[17] Jahnsen FL, Moloney ED, Hogan T, et al. Rapid dendritic cell recruitment to the bronchial mucosa of patients with atopic asthma in response to local allergen challenge. Thorax 2001; 56:823–6.
[18] Bertorelli G, Bocchino V, Zhou X, et al. Dendritic cell number is related to IL-4 expression in the airways of atopic asthmatic subjects. Allergy 2000;55:449–54.
[19] Agea E, Forenza N, Piattoni S, et al. Expression of B7 co-stimulatory molecules and CD1a antigen by alveolar macrophages in allergic bronchial asthma. Clin Exp Allergy 1998;28: 1359–67.
[20] Agea E, Bistoni O, Russano AM, et al. The biology of cypress allergy. Allergy 2002;57: 959–60.
[21] Agiular L, Ortega-Pierresi G, Campos B, et al. Phospholipid membranes form specific nonbilayer molecular arrangements that are antigenic. J Biol Chem 1999;274:25193–6.
[22] Agea E, Russano A, Bistoni O, et al. Human CD1-restricted recognition of lipids from pollens. J Exp Med 2005;202:295–308.
[23] Baeza I, Wong C, Mondragon R, et al. Transbilayer diffusion of divalent cations mediated by phosphatidate particles. J Mol Evol 1994;39:560–8.
[24] Kobayashi E, Motoki K, Uchida T, et al. KRN7000, a novel immunomodulator, and its antitumor activity. Oncol Res 1995;7:529–34.
[25] Rauch J, Gumperz J, Robinson C, et al. Structural features of the acyl chain determine self-phospholipid antigen recognition by a CD1d-restricted invariant NKT cell. J Biol Chem 2003;278:47508–15.
[26] Akbari O. The role of iNKT cells in development of bronchial asthma: a translational approach from animal models to human. Allergy 2006;67:962–8.
[27] Russano AM, Agea E, Corazzi L, et al. Recognition of pollen-derived phosphatidyl-ethanolamine by human CD1d-restricted γδ T cells. J Allergy Clin Immunol 2006;117:1178–84.
[28] Heeley EL, Hohlfeld JM, Krug N, et al. Phospholipid molecular species of bronchoalveolar lavage fluid after local allergen challenge in asthma. Am J Physiol Lung Cell Mol Physiol 2000;278:L305–11.
[29] Wright SM, Hockey PM, Enhorning G, et al. Altered airway surfactant phospholipid composition and reduced lung function in asthma. J Appl Physiol 2000;89:1283–92.
[30] Busse WW, Coffman RL, Gelfand EW, et al. Mechanisms of persistent airway inflammation in asthma. A role for T cells and T-cell products. Am J Respir Crit Care Med 1995;152: 388–93.
[31] Erpenbeck VJ, Agenberg A, Dulkys Y, et al. Natural porcine surfactant augments airway inflammation after allergen challenge in patients with asthma. Am J Respir Crit Care Med 2004;169:578–86.
[32] Lisbonne M, Diem S, de Castro KA, et al. Cutting edge: invariant Valpha14 NKT cells are required for allergen-induced airway inflammation and hyperreactivity in an experimental asthma model. J Immunol 2003;171:1637–41.
[33] Araujo LM, Lefort J, Nahori MA, et al. Exacerbated Th2-mediated airway inflammation and hyperresponsiveness in autoimmune diabetes-prone NOD mice: a critical role for CD1d-dependent NKT cells. Eur J Immunol 2004;34:327–35.
[34] Hachem P, Lisbonne M, Michel ML, et al. Alpha-galactosyl-ceramide-induced iNKT cells suppress experimental allergic asthma in sensitized mice: role of IFN-gamma. Eur J Immunol 2005;35:2793–802.
[35] Uldrich AP, Crowe NY, Kyparissoudis K, et al. NKT cell stimulation with glycolipid antigen in vivo: costimulation-dependent expansion, Bim-dependent contraction, and hyporesponsiveness to further antigenic challenge. J Immunol 2005;175:3092–101.

[36] Pham-Thi N, de Blic J, Le Bourgeois M, et al. Enhanced frequency of immunoregulatory invariant natural killer T cells in the airways of children with asthma. J Allergy Clin Immunol 2006;117:217–8.

[37] Akbari O, Faul JL, Hoyte EG, et al. CD4+ invariant T-cell-receptor+ natural killer T cells in bronchial asthma. N Engl J Med 2006;354:1117–29.

[38] Thomas SY, Lilly CM, Luster AD. Invariant natural killer T cells in bronchial asthma. N Engl J Med 2006;354:2613–5.

[39] Spinozzi F, Agea E, Bistoni O, et al. γδ T cells, allergen recognition and airway inflammation. Immunol Today 1998;219:22–6.

[40] Morita CT, Mariuzza RA, Brenner MB. Antigen recognition by human γδ T cells: pattern recognition by the adaptive immune system. Springer Semin Immunopathol 2000;22:191–217.

[41] Augustin A, Kubo RT, Sim G-K. Resident pulmonary lymphocytes express the γδ T cell receptor. Nature 1989;340:239–41.

[42] McMenamin C, Pimm C, McKersey M, et al. Regulation of IgE responses to inhaled antigen in mice by antigen-specific γδ T cells. Science 1994;265:1869–71.

[43] Gascan H, Aversa GG, Gauchat J-F, et al. Membranes of activated CD4+ T cells expressing T cell receptor (TcR) alpha beta or TcR gamma delta induce IgE synthesis by human B cells in the presence of interleukin-4. Eur J Immunol 1992;22:1133–41.

[44] Okuda M, Pawankar R. Flow cytometric analysis of intraepithelial lymphocytes in the human nasal mucosa. Allergy 1992;47:255–9.

[45] Spinozzi F, Agea E, Bistoni O, et al. Increased allergen-specific, steroid-sensitive γδ T cells in bronchoalveolar lavage fluid from patients with asthma. Ann Intern Med 1996;124:223–7.

[46] Spinozzi F, Agea E, Bistoni O, et al. Local expansion of allergen-specific CD30+ Th2-type γδ T cells in bronchial asthma. Mol Med 1995;1:821–6.

[47] Moody DB, Ulrichs T, Muhlecker W, et al. CD1c-mediated T cell recognition of isoprenoid glycolipids in *Mycobacterium tuberculosis* infection. Nature 2000;404:884–8.

[48] Willis-Karp M. Immunologic basis of antigen-induced airway hyperresponsiveness. Annu Rev Immunol 1999;17:255–81.

[49] Trottein F, Mallevaey T, Faveeuw C, et al. Role of the natural killer T lymphocytes in Th2 responses during allergic asthma and helminth parasitic diseases. Chem Immunol Allergy 2006;90:113–27.

[50] Akbari O, Stock P, Umetsu DT. Role of regulatory T cells in allergy and asthma. Curr Opin Immunol 2003;15:627–33.

ELSEVIER
SAUNDERS

Immunol Allergy Clin N Am
27 (2007) 93–103

IMMUNOLOGY
AND ALLERGY
CLINICS
OF NORTH AMERICA

Chimeric Human Fcγ–Allergen Fusion Proteins in the Prevention of Allergy

Ke Zhang, MD, PhD[a,*], Daocheng Zhu, PhD[b], Christopher Kepley, PhD[c], Tetsuya Terada, MD, PhD[a,d], Andrew Saxon, MD[a]

[a]*The Hart and Louise Lyon Laboratory, Division of Clinical Immunology/Allergy, Department of Medicine, UCLA School of Medicine, 52-175 CHS, 10833 Le Conte Avenue, Los Angeles, CA 90095-1680, USA*

[b]*Division of Allergy-Immunology, Department of Medicine, M-215, Northwestern University, 240 East Huron Street, Chicago, IL 60611, USA*

[c]*Division of Rheumatology, Allergy and Immunology, Department of Internal Medicine, Virginia Commonwealth University Health System, 1112 Clay Street, Richmond, VA 23298-0263, USA*

[d]*Department of Otorhinolaryngology, Osaka Medical College, 2-7 Daigaku-cho, Takatsuki, Osaka 569-8686, Japan*

Allergic responses are strongly associated with Th2-type immune responses, and modulation of the skewed Th2 response toward a more balanced response is the major goal of allergen immunotherapy (IT) in allergic disorders. To achieve this goal, several approaches have been tested, including allergen protein-, peptide-, modified allergen protein–, and allergy gene–based IT [1–3]. Traditionally, allergen IT has relied on the frequent injection of gradually escalated amounts of extracted allergen proteins. However, even when given according to a cautious and protracted schedule, standard allergen IT causes local and systemic allergic reactions and may elicit rare but life-threatening reactions [4,5]. Therefore, investigators have great interest in developing novel forms of allergen IT in terms of safety and efficacy. The authors have shown that a human immunoglobulin (Ig) Fcγ–Fcϵ fusion protein (GE2) that directly cross-links the high-affinity IgE receptors (FcϵRI) and low-affinity IgG receptors (FcγRIIb) on human

Supported by an USPHS-NIH grant AI-15251 to Andrew Saxon, MD.

* Corresponding author.
E-mail address: kzhang@mednet.ucla.edu (K. Zhang).

doi:10.1016/j.iac.2006.11.002
immunology.theclinics.com

mast cells and basophils was able to inhibit degranulation [6], they reasoned that human gamma–allergen fusion protein would achieve a similar inhibitory effect in an allergen-specific fashion while preserving the immunogenicity of the allergen component. Therefore, the authors constructed and developed a human–cat chimeric fusion protein composed of the human Fcγ1 and the cat allergen Fel d1 (*Felis domesticus*) for cat allergen–specific IT [7,8]. This article summarizes the therapeutic features and potential of this novel fusion protein for allergic IT.

Role of FcγRIIb in inhibiting allergic response

Cross-linking of the high-affinity IgE receptor (FcεRI) activates tyrosine phosphorylation of immunoreceptor tyrosine–based activation motifs (ITAMs) in the β and γ subunits of FcεRI in the cytoplasmic tails and leads to cell activation and degranulation in basophils and mast cells [4,5]. This process leads to the classic immediate hypersensitivity reaction. The activation signal is balanced by the inhibitory receptors on these cells [9]. Human mast cells and basophils express the low-affinity IgG receptor (FcγRIIb), which contains an immunoreceptor tyrosine–based inhibitory motif (ITIMs) within its cytoplasmic tail [9]. Coaggregation of FcεRI to FcγRIIb has been shown to block in vitro and in vivo human basophil and mast cell function [10–13]. This inhibition is mediated through reduction in tyrosine phosphorylation of Syk, ERK, and several other cellular substrates, and increased tyrosine phosphorylation of the adapter protein downstream of kinase (Dok), growth factor receptor–bound protein 2 (Grb2), and SH2 domain containing inositol 5-phosphatase (SHIP) [8,14]. A previously developed Fcγ–Fcε fusion protein, GE2 [6], exhibited its inhibitory role in allergic responses in an allergen-nonspecific manner through directly cross-linking the FcεRI and FcγRIIb on mast cells and basophils. A more detailed review of this subject was published elsewhere [15].

Fcγ–Fel d1 fusion protein inhibits Fel d1–mediated allergic degranulation

To explore whether allergic responses can be modified in an allergen-specific manner through indirect co–cross-linking of the FcγRIIb and FcεRI bound the allergen-specific IgE, the authors genetically linked an allergen molecule using a flexible linker to a human Fcγ region. Because Fel d1 is the dominant allergen for cat allergy, and cat allergy is a major clinical problem, the authors constructed a chimeric human–cat protein composed of the hinge-through-CH_3 portion of human IgGγ1 Fc region fused to Fel d1 [7].

To test the efficacy of a chimeric human–cat fusion protein (GFD) on degranulation, freshly purified human basophils were purified from patients who had cat allergy, and were cultured along with various doses of GFD ranging from 1 ng/mL to 1 μg/mL, followed by the challenge with an optimal dose of purified Fel d1. GFD at 10 ng/mL inhibited histamine release by more than 75% ($P<.002$), whereas at 100 ng/mL, inhibition reached more than 90% ($P<.001$) (Fig. 1A). Similar inhibition was observed in cord blood–derived mast cells sensitized with cat-allergic serum. At 10 μg/mL, GFD reduced FcεRI-mediated release by an average of 77% ($P<.05$) in a dose-dependent fashion (Fig. 1B). Critically, these results also showed that GFD does not function as an allergen because prerelease of mediators was not observed when Fel d1–sensitized basophils were incubated with GFD. These results indicated that GFD was able to block the Fel d1-induced degranulation of human mast cells and basophils, and that fusion of Fel d1 to the Fcγ altered the allergen nature of the Fel d1.

Fcγ–Fel d1 fusion protein inhibits signal events associated with degranulation

Tyrosine phosphorylation is a key event connecting FcεRI cross-linking to downstream signaling in human mast cells and basophils. Previous investigations have shown that the mitogen-activated protein (MAP) kinases ERK1/2 and Syk are quickly phosphorylated in IgE-stimulated human FcεRI–positive cells [16,17]. To determine whether GFD is able to alter these critical early signaling events responsible for the early activation of mast cells and basophils, the authors investigated the role of GFD in IgE-dependent, FcεRI-mediated kinase phosphorylations. Cross-linking FcεRI on cord blood mast cells with IgE directed to Fel d1 induces substantial tyrosine phosphorylation of Syk and ERK, which was markedly reduced in cells preincubated with GFD (Fig. 2). Inhibition was observed 2 minutes after antigen stimulation and persisted as long as 15 minutes. Therefore, GFD coaggregation of FcεRI and FcγRII through formation of a Fcγ–Fel d1–IgE complex inhibits IgE-mediated Syk and ERK phosphorylation and is probably responsible for inhibiting basophil and mast cell function.

Fcγ–Fel d1 fusion protein blocks passive cutaneous anaphylaxis reaction in FcεRIα transgenic mice

Allergic degranulation of mast cells in vivo can be determined with a passive cutaneous anaphylaxis (PCA) assay in transgenic (Tg) mice expressing human FcεRIα [6,7]. After the back skin of the FcεRIα Tg mice is passively sensitized with human IgE from patients who have cat allergy and the mice undergo subsequent challenge with the appropriate antigen, results of the PCA are positive. Because the mast cells in these Tg mice also express the murine FcγRIIb that binds to human IgG [6], the inhibitory effects of GFD through co-crosslinking the humanized FcεRI and murine FcγRIIb can be tested using this PCA model.

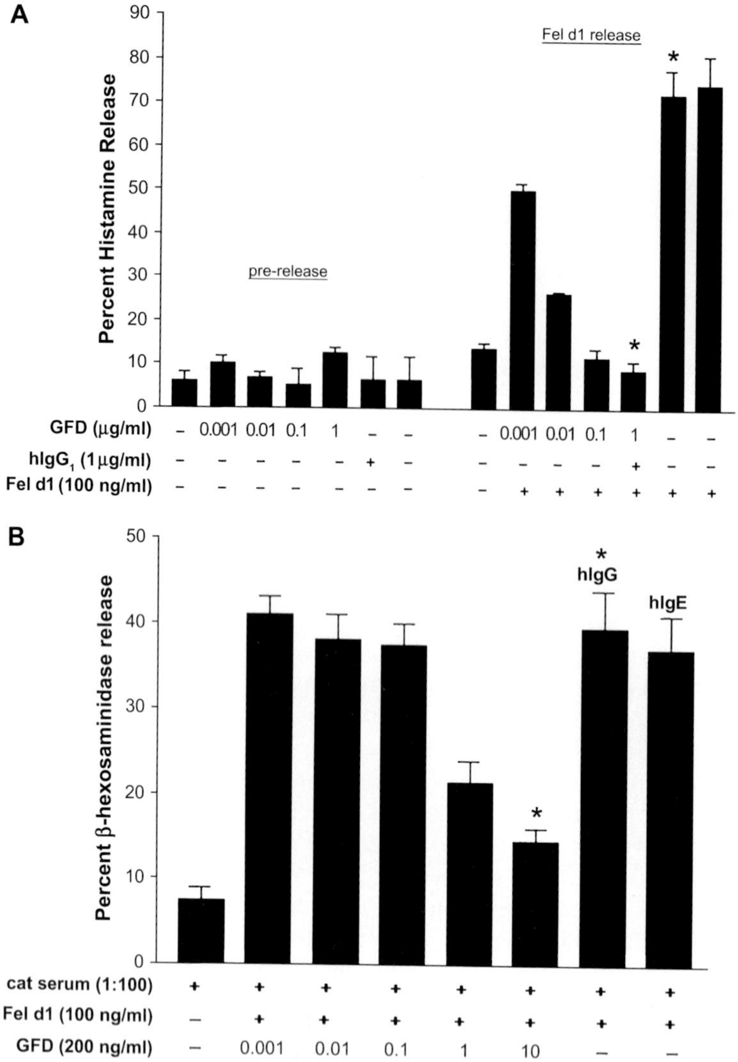

Fig. 1. GFD inhibits fresh human basophil and mast cell degranulation. (*A*) Dose-dependent inhibition of basophil histamine release by GFD. Basophils from an atopic donor were incubated for 2 hours with GFD and the supernatant assayed for histamine (pre-release). Cells were washed and then challenged with Fel d1 and histamine was measured in the supernatant (Fel d1 release). (*B*) Dose-dependent inhibition of fresh cord blood-derived mast cell β-hexosaminidase release using GFD. The results from one experiment, performed in duplicate, are representative of three separate donors. The asterisk indicates a statistically significant difference when comparing the two conditions. Human IgG and IgE are represented as hIgG and hIgE, respectively. (*Adapted from* Zhu D, Kepley CL, Zhang K, et al. A chimeric human–cat fusion protein blocks cat-induced allergy. Nat Med 2005;11:446–9; with permission.)

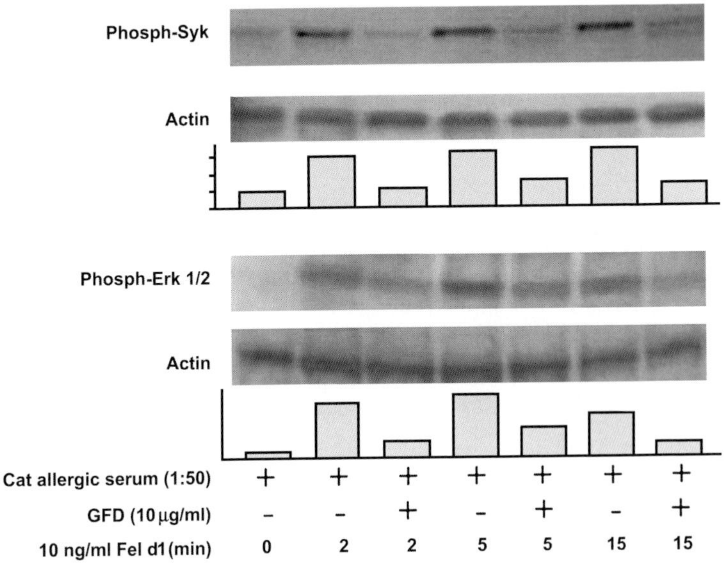

Fig. 2. GFD inhibits FcεRI-mediated Syk and ERK phosphorylation. Cord blood–derived mast cells were sensitized with cat-allergic serum, washed, and Western blotted with the indicated antibodies. Results are representative of three separate experiments. (*Adapted from* Zhu D, Kepley CL, Zhang K, et al. A chimeric human–cat fusion protein blocks cat-induced allergy. Nat Med 2005;11:446–9, with permission.)

As shown in Fig. 3A, GFD inhibited the IgE-mediated PCA of a patient allergic to cats in a dose-dependent manner (panel I–IV), and GFD at 100 ng per spot completely blocked the PCA (panel IV). Analogous inhibition was also observed by using GE2 fusion protein (Fig. 3B). However, GFD exhibited higher efficacy for blocking PCA reactivity compared with GE2 (see Fig. 3B), with at least tenfold less amounts of GFD required for complete blocking of PCA (see Fig. 3B, panels III versus IV). GFD blocked PCA reactivity equally well when injected 4 hours after or simultaneously with the serum of a patient who had cat allergy (see Fig. 3B, panel III versus II). The purified IgE-dependent PCA of the patient who had a cat allergy, as shown by the inactivation of the PCA activity by heating the IgE with 56°C for 30 minutes [18], was also completely blocked by GFD. As a specificity control, GFD did not inhibit PCA reactivity to the human anti-NP (4-hydroxy-3-nitrophenylacetyl) IgE (data not shown). GFD itself was not inducing mast cell release at sensitized sites (data not shown). These data showed that GFD is able to block the Fel d1 allergen–specific allergic response in vivo.

Fcγ–Fel d1 fusion protein blocks the allergic responses in a mouse model

A Balb/c mouse model of systemic reactivity to Fel d1 in actively sensitized mice was used to test the immunotherapeutic ability of GFD. The

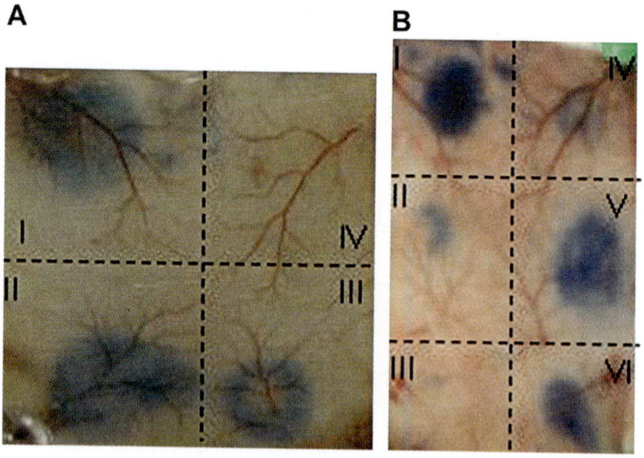

Fig. 3. In vivo GFD inhibits IgE-mediated degranulation in transgenic mice expressing human FcεRIα. (*A*) Dose-dependent inhibition of PCA by GFD. The labeled back skin sites were sensitized with cat-allergic serum (1:5 dilution) for 4 hours, followed by the administration of (I) saline; (II) 1 ng of GFD in 50 μL saline; (III) 10 ng of GFD; and (IV) 100 ng of GFD. (*B*) Comparison of GFD and GE2 for their ability to inhibit PCA reactivity to human anti–Fel d1 IgE. The skin sites were sensitized with 1:5 diluted cat-allergic serum, with the following treatment: (I) saline injection 4 hours later; (II) 100 ng GFD 4 hours later; (II) 100 ng GFD simultaneously with serum; (IV) 1 μg GE2 simultaneously with serum; (V) 100 ng GE2 4 hours later; and (VI) 100 ng GE2 simultaneously with serum. (*Adapted from* Zhu D, Kepley CL, Zhang K, et al. A chimeric human–cat fusion protein blocks cat-induced allergy. Nat Med 2005;11:446–9; with permission.)

rationale for this murine model to test the effects of human IgG Fc–Fel d1 fusion protein GFD is based on the fact that the murine Fc receptors for IgG (FcγRs) will bind human IgG Fc [13]. Thus, the Fc portion of GFD is expected to bind murine FcγRs, including FcγRIIb, which contains the ITIM that drives inhibitory signaling. The Fel d1 portion of GFD will also bind to murine Fel d1–specific IgE or IgG1 on the surface of sensitized mast cells and basophils.

BALB/c mice were sensitized with Fed d1 and treated according to the protocol diagrammed in Fig. 4A. The core body temperature, which was used as the indicator for systemic anaphylaxis, dropped by an average of 1.7°C ± 0.2°C starting at 5 minutes after the challenge (Fig. 4D). This decreased body temperature was completely blocked by the GFD treatment ($P<.001$). GFD treatment also completely blocked Fel d1–induced airway hyperresponsiveness (AHR) (Fig. 4B), as assessed through pulmonary resistance after methacholine challenge. Similarly, the eosinophilic airway inflammation in Fel d1–sensitized and intratracheally challenged mice, which was evident through increased eosinophils in bronchoalveolar lavage fluid, was blunted by GFD treatment (Fig. 4C). These results indicate that allergic responses to Fel d1 could be ameliorated by GFD treatment and these beneficial immunomodulatory effects occurred when GFD was

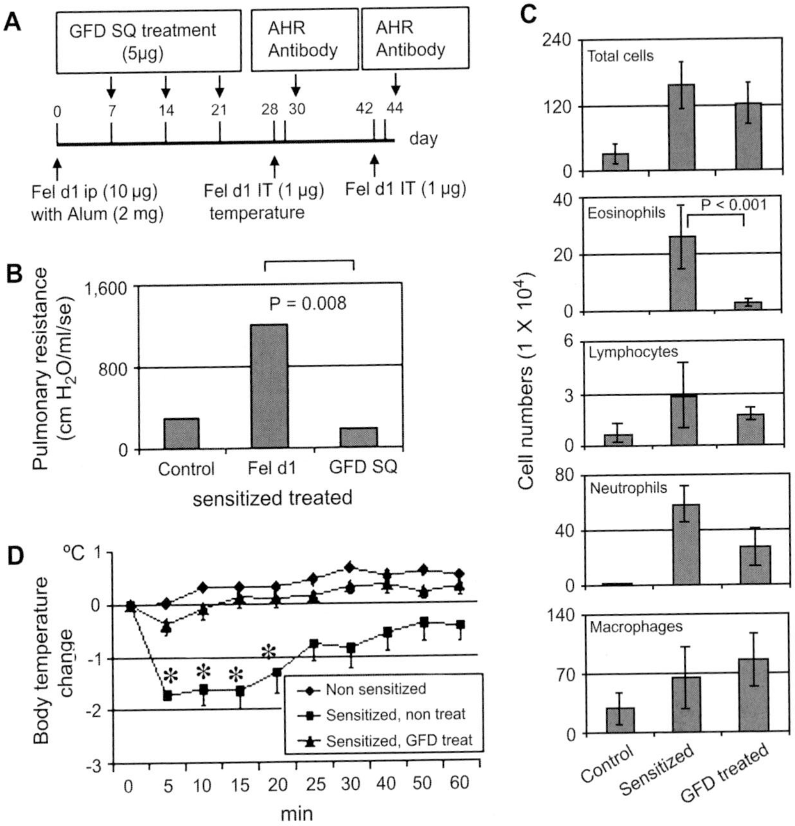

Fig. 4. Subcutaneous (SQ) administration of GFD blocked Fel d1–induced allergic response in a mouse model. (*A*) Schematic diagram of the experimental protocol. (*B*) Effect of GFD on blocking Fel d1–induced systemic allergic reactivity. The body temperature changes were assessed immediately after Fel d1 IT challenge (1 μg) with 5-minute intervals. The asterisk indicates a statistically significant difference between the two conditions. (*C*) Effect of GFD on Fel d1–induced AHR. The airway resistance to methacholine challenge was assessed using a computer-controlled small-animal FlexiVent® ventilator 2 days after IT Fel d1 challenge. The numbers represent the average values from three measurements of the airway resistance from a group of mice for each condition. (*D*) Effect of GFD on Fel d1–induced pulmonary eosinophilic inflammation. Total and differential numbers of bronchoalveolar lavage fluid cells were counted. (*Adapted from* Zhu D, Kepley CL, Zhang K, et al. A chimeric human–cat fusion protein blocks cat-induced allergy. Nat Med 2005;11:446–9; with permission.)

administrated in a regimen similar to allergen IT after initial allergen sensitization. Anti–Fel d1 IgG1, IgG2a, and IgE responses induced by Fel d1 immunization showed variable changes in response to GFD treatment, but these changes did not reach statistical significance (data not shown). These results indicated that a protocol of allergen IT significantly inhibited allergic response to Fel d1 in a mouse model.

Fcγ–Fel d1 fusion protein fails to induce local or systemic reactivity on administration to Fel d1–sensitized animals

Because GFD is a fusion protein containing Fel d1, whether GFD itself would function as Fel d1 to induce allergic reactivity was important to determine. The authors undertook several approaches to examine this issue. As shown in Fig. 1A, GFD alone was not able to mediate histamine release from human basophils of patients who had cat allergy. In Fel d1–sensitized mice, Fel d1 induced a systemic allergic reactivity as shown through significant body temperature reduction (2.58°C ± 0.4°C). In contrast, an equimolar amount of GFD did not induce a significant temperature reduction in sensitized animals. In addition, IT administration of GFD did not induce AHR, as was seen with Fel d1. Intradermal injection of Fel d1 induced mast cell degranulation in the skin of Fel d1–sensitized BALB/c mice, but GFD did not induce the skin reactivity in sensitized animals. These data strongly indicated that GFD failed to elicit allergic reactivity systemically in the skin or airways of Fel d1–sensitized animals.

Fcγ–Fel d1 fusion protein blocks Fel d1–induced allergic reactivity in rush immunotherapy settings

Using the experimental regimen capable of blocking Fel d1–mediated allergic responses in a BALB/c mice model, the authors further sought to test whether GFD, when administered in a protocol to mimic rush IT (eg, high-dose GFD administrated in a short period), was able to inhibit Fel d1-dependent allergic responses in already highly sensitized animals, and whether a single administration of GFD was sufficient to acutely block reactivity in animals with established Fel d1–induced allergic responses.

The Fel d1–induced systemic reaction, measured using core temperature changes, was inhibited for a longer duration in the rush IT setting in which GFD was administered three times, whereas only acute, but not delayed, systemic reaction was inhibited by the single administration of GFD [8], in a similar manner as shown in Fig. 4D. Administration of GFD as the rush IT in the sensitized mice also blocked skin mast cell degranulation, assayed using an active skin test [8].

Fel d1–induced airway responsiveness and allergic lung inflammation were blocked by the rush IT protocols. Treatment with GFD completely reversed the Fel d1–induced airway hyperresponsiveness to methacholine and blunted the airway allergic inflammation, as shown through the significantly decrease either in the percentage or absolute numbers of eosinophils in the bronchoalveolar lavage fluid ($P<.001$). Histologic examination showed that Fel d1-induced pulmonary inflammation (Fig. 5A) was significantly inhibited by GFD administration ($P<.001$) (Fig. 5B). Marked goblet cell metaplasia was observed in the large airways of sensitized mice and Fel d1–treated mice, whereas GFD treatment inhibited this goblet cell metaplasia (Fig. 5C). These

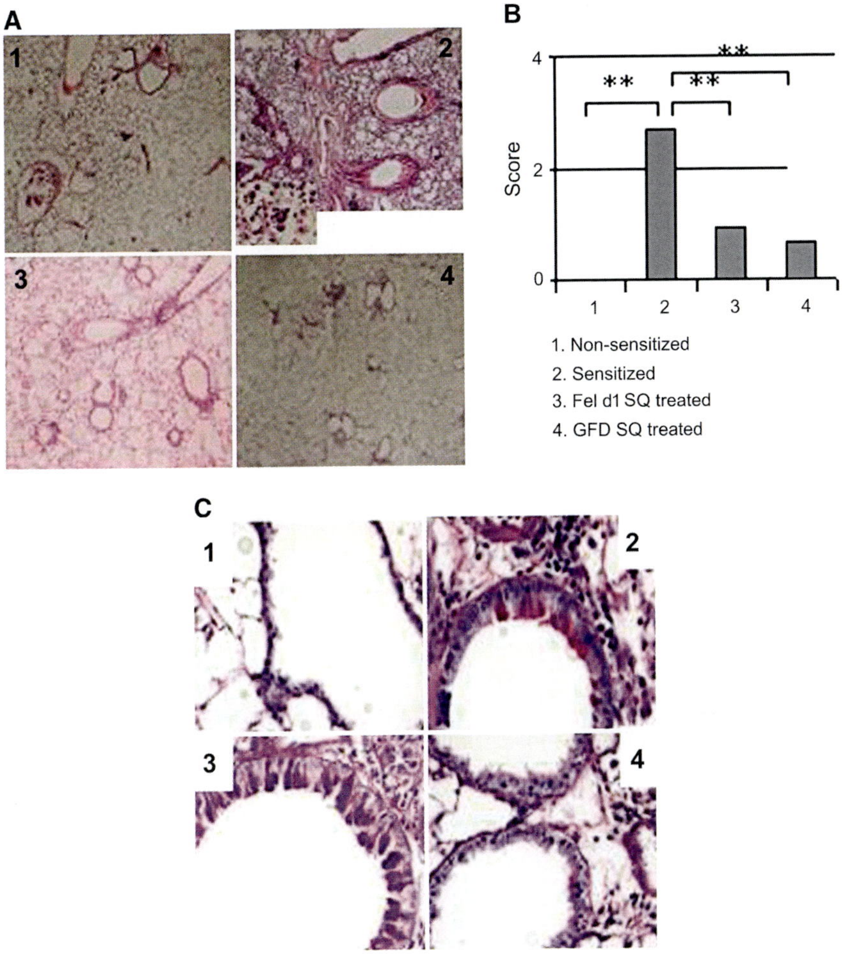

Fig. 5. Lung histologic changes in GFD–treated mice. (*A*) Light photomicrographs of hematoxylin and eosin–stained sections of lung tissue from the different treatments. Few leukocytes were observed in the lung of nonsensitized mice (*panel 1*). In contrast, numerous eosinophils were present after Fel d1 challenge in the control mice (*panel 2*). Both Fel d1 and GFD treatments (*panels 3 and 4*) led to markedly decreased eosinophil accumulation in the lung. (*B*) Semi-quantitative analysis of the eosinophil accumulation in the lungs of animals challenged with IT with Fel d1 at day 54. Results of each group are expressed as mean ± SD. The asterisks indicate $P < .001$ between the groups. (*C*) Light photomicrographs of periodic acid-Schiff–stained sections of lung tissue from nonsensitized mice (*panel 1*) and mice receiving the different treatments. Marked goblet cell metaplasia was observed in large airways in the sensitized–challenged animals (*panel 2*). GFD treatment (*panel 4*), but not Fel d1 (*panel 3*), clearly inhibited this goblet cell metaplasia (*Adapted from* Terada T, Zhang K, Belperio J, et al. A chimeric human-cat Fcgamma-Fel d1 fusion protein inhibits systemic, pulmonary, and cutaneous allergic reactivity to intratracheal challenge in mice sensitized to Fel d1, the major cat allergen. Clin Immunol 2006;120:45–56; with permission.)

results indicted that Fel d1–induced allergic responses were significantly blocked by the rush IT protocol with higher-dose GFD administration.

Fcγ–Fel d1 fusion protein immunotherapy modulates the antibody response to Fel d1

To examine whether the administration of GFD with rush IT protocol was able to modulate the antibody responses to Fel d1, the Fel d1–specific IgG1, IgG2a, and IgE were analyzed. The Fel d1 sensitization and challenge induced significant increases in serum Fel d1 antibodies, with levels ranging from undetectable (<1.0 U/mL) for nonsensitized animals to geometric means of 57,859, 2, and 113 U/mL for IgG1, IgE, and IgG2, respectively ($P<.01$ for all), reflecting the Th2–dominant allergic antibody responses. GFD treatment led to increased IgG1 antibodies to Fel d1 compared with untreated (geometric means of 186,167 versus 57,859 U/mL; $P<.05$) and Fel d1–treated animals (186,167 versus 33,157 U/mL; $P<.02$). GFD did not alter IgE or IgG2 antibodies (geometric means of 34.4 and 166 U/mL, respectively) and Fel d1 treatment did not significantly alter any antibodies levels (geometric means of 33,157, 14.2, and 140 U/mL for IgG1, IgE, and IgG2a, respectively) compared with untreated animals.

Potential use of Fcγ–Fel d1 fusion protein for allergic blockade and immunotherapy in cat allergy

Data show that the chimeric GFD protein is a promising model for a new form of IT in allergy and a specific intervention against cat allergy. The advantages of this approach are that the allergen carries its own negative signal, the Fcγ portion that has been shown to drive inhibitory signaling in human mast cells and basophils. GFD's indirect cross-linking of FcγRIIb and FcεRI through naturally occurring IgE to Fel d1 results in an acute antigen–specific inhibition of mediator release. As a result, from a safety perspective, GFD should be able to be given safely in high doses and a much briefer timeframe than conventional immunotherapy, with the only limitation being the time and dose necessary to induce the desired beneficial long-term modulation of the individual's allergic response to cats. If successful, a similar approach could be undertaken in severe food allergy, where many of the specific allergens are known and therapeutic options are severely limited.

References

[1] Palmer K, Burks W. Current developments in peanut allergy. Curr Opin Allergy Clin Immunol 2006;6:202–6.

[2] Ferreira F, Briza P, Infuhr D, et al. Modified recombinant allergens for safer immunotherapy. Inflamm Allergy Drug Targets 2006;5:5–14.

[3] Raz E, Tighe H, Sato Y, et al. Preferential induction of a Th_1 immune response and inhibition of specific IgE antibody formation by plasmid DNA immunization. Proc Natl Acad Sci U S A 1996;93:5141–5.
[4] Oliver JM, Kepley CL, Ortega E, et al. Immunologically mediated signaling in basophils and mast cells: finding therapeutic targets for allergic diseases in the human FcεRI signaling pathway. Immunopharmacology 2000;48:269–81.
[5] Daeron M. Fc receptor biology. Annu Rev Immunol 1997;15:203–34.
[6] Zhu D, Kepley CL, Zhang M, et al. A novel human immunoglobulin Fcγ-Fcε bifunctional fusion protein inhibits FcεRI-mediated degranulation. Nat Med 2002;8:518–21.
[7] Zhu D, Kepley CL, Zhang K, et al. A chimeric human–cat fusion protein blocks cat-induced allergy. Nat Med 2005;11:446–9.
[8] Terada T, Zhang K, Belperio J, et al. A chimeric human-cat Fcgamma-Fel d1 fusion protein inhibits systemic, pulmonary, and cutaneous allergic reactivity to intratracheal challenge in mice sensitized to Fel d1, the major cat allergen. Clin Immunol 2006;120:45–56.
[9] Malbec O, Fong DC, Turner M, et al. Fcε Receptor I-associated lyn-dependent phosphorylation of Fcγ Receptor IIB during negative regulation of mast cell activation. J Immunol 1998;160:1647–58.
[10] Fong DC, Malbec O, Arock M, et al. Selective in vivo recruitment of the phosphatidylinositol phosphatase SHIP by phosphorylated FcγR IIB during negative regulation of IgE-dependent mouse mast cell activation. Immunol Lett 1996;54:83–91.
[11] Ott VL, Cambier JC. Activating and inhibitory signaling in mast cells: new opportunities for therapeutic intervention? J Allergy Clin Immunol 2000;106:429–40.
[12] Ono M, Bolland S, Tempst P, et al. Role of the inositol phosphatase SHIP in negative regulation of the immune system by the receptor FcγRIIB. Nature 1996;383:263–6.
[13] Tam SW, Demissie S, Thomas D, et al. A bispecific antibody against human IgE and human FcgammaRII that inhibits antigen-induced histamine release by human mast cells and basophils. Allergy 2004;59:772–80.
[14] Kepley CL, Taghavi S, Mackay G, et al. Co-aggregation of FcγRII with FcεRI on human mast cells inhibits antigen-induced secretion and involves SHIP-Grb2-Dok complexes. J Biol Chem 2004;279:35139–49.
[15] Saxon A, Zhu D, Zhang K, et al. Genetically engineered negative signaling molecules in the immunomodulation of allergic diseases. Curr Opin Allergy Clin Immunol 2004;4:563–8.
[16] Daeron M, Malbec O, Latour S, et al. Regulation of high-affinity IgE receptor-mediated mast cell activation by murine low-affinity IgG receptors. J Clin Invest 1995;95:577–85.
[17] Suzuki H, Takei M, Yanagida M, et al. Early and late events in Fc epsilon RI signal transduction in human cultured mast cells. J Immunol 1997;159:5881–8.
[18] Zhang K, Kepley CL, Terada T, et al. Inhibition of allergen-specific IgE reactivity by a human Ig Fcγ-Fcε bifunctional protein. J Allergy Clin Immunol 2004;114:321–7.

ELSEVIER
SAUNDERS

Immunol Allergy Clin N Am
27 (2007) 105–127

IMMUNOLOGY
AND ALLERGY
CLINICS
OF NORTH AMERICA

New Perspectives for Use of Native and Engineered Recombinant Food Proteins in Treatment of Food Allergy

Anna Nowak-Wegrzyn, MD

Jaffe Food Allergy Institute, Division of Allergy and Immunology, Department of Pediatrics, Mount Sinai School of Medicine, Box 1198, One G. Levy Place, NY 10029, USA

Food allergy is defined as an adverse reaction to food mediated by the immune system [1]. Food allergies affect 2% to 4% of adults and 6% to 8% of young children in westernized societies [2]. An estimated 12 million of Americans, including 2 million school-aged children, have food allergy. Food allergic reactions account for approximately 30,000 emergency room visits, and severe food anaphylaxis is implicated in 150 to 200 deaths per year in the United States [3]. Cow's milk, egg white, soybean, wheat, peanut, tree nuts, and fish are responsible for more than 90% of food allergies in children. In adults, peanut, tree nuts, shellfish, and fish are implicated in most severe reactions, whereas the most common food allergens are fruits and vegetables that cause oral pruritus in persons with respiratory pollen allergy [4–7]. Most childhood food allergies to cow's milk, egg white, soybean, and wheat resolve with time, whereas peanut, tree nut, fish, and shellfish allergies tend to be life-long conditions [8–10].

Diagnosis of food allergy relies on a detailed history, including type of food, amount ingested, and timing and severity of symptoms, and laboratory diagnostic tests for detecting food allergen–specific IgE antibody in the skin (using a skin prick test) or in serum (preferably using ImmunoCAP). A double-blind, placebo-controlled oral food challenge is the current gold standard for diagnosing food allergy [1,11]. Feeding the suspected food under physician supervision is indicated in an individual who has no recent (past 6–12 months) history of convincing reactions and whose laboratory

Funding support: K23AI059318 to A. Nowak-Wegrzyn.
E-mail address: anna.nowak-wegrzyn@mssm.edu

doi:10.1016/j.iac.2006.11.006 ***immunology.theclinics.com***

tests are below the high predictive value for clinical reactivity (Fig. 1) [12,13]. Management of food allergy requires dietary avoidance of the implicated foods and prompt treatment of allergic reactions. Accidental food allergic reactions are very common; despite avoidance, one study showed that

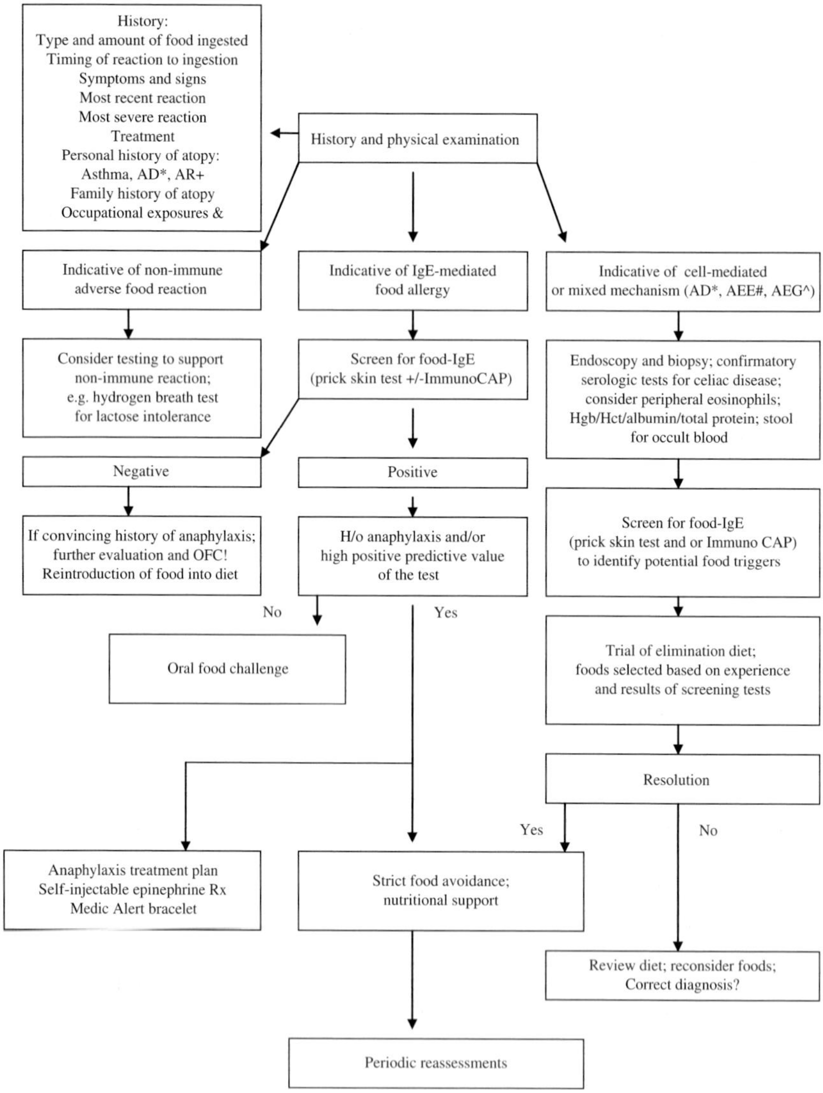

Fig. 1. A scheme of current approach to diagnosis and management of food allergy. AD*, atopic dermatitis; AR+, allergic rhinitis and occupational exposures to inhaled food dust important in bakers and millers with asthma; AEE#, allergic eosinophilic esophagitis; AEGˆ, allergic eosinophilic gastroenteritis; OFC!, oral food challenge.

approximately 50% of children who had peanut allergies experienced at least one accidental reaction to peanut over a 2-year period [14].

Recent epidemiologic data indicate that prevalence of peanut allergy doubled in the past 5 to 10 years in the United States, the United Kingdom, and Canada [4,5,15,16]. Currently, peanut allergy affects approximately 1% of young children, most (80%) of whom will have lifelong peanut allergy [8]. Peanut was identified as the food allergen responsible for most severe and fatal food anaphylactic reactions in the United States [17]. The reasons why peanut allergy prevalence is increasing are unknown, but considering rapid changes, environmental factors seem to play a more significant role than genetic factors. Current prevention guidelines that recommend delaying introduction of dietary peanut until age 3 years to children at risk for atopy have not been effective in decreasing the risk for peanut allergy [18].

Considering the above factors, food allergy emerged as an important target for research on curative treatment and prevention, with most efforts focusing on peanut, cow's milk, and egg allergy. This article reviews the recent developments in potential treatments for IgE-mediated food allergy using native and engineered recombinant food proteins.

Immunotherapy with native food proteins

Subcutaneous peanut immunotherapy

Subcutaneous allergen immunotherapy is used as standard and effective treatment for allergic rhinitis, asthma, and venom allergy [19]. Subcutaneous immunotherapy with peanut extract has been studied in a small number of individuals who had peanut allergy. One double-blind, placebo-controlled study treated individuals who had confirmed peanut allergy with peanut immunotherapy or placebo [20]. Objective measures of efficacy included changes in symptom score during double-blind placebo-controlled food challenge (DBPCFC) to peanut and titrated end point skin prick tests (SPT). Three subjects treated with peanut immunotherapy completed the study. These subjects showed a 67% to 100% decrease in symptoms evaluated by DBPCFC and showed a 2- to 5-log reduction in end point SPT reactivity to peanut extract. One subject treated with placebo completed the study. This subject had essentially no change in DBPCFC symptom scores or SPT sensitivity to peanut. Two other subjects treated with placebo underwent a second SPT. These subjects experienced a 1- to 2-log increase in skin test sensitivity to peanut. All subjects treated with peanut immunotherapy reached maintenance dose, and the rate of systemic reactions with rush immunotherapy was 13.3%. Because of a tragic pharmacy error, one control patient in the placebo group died of anaphylactic shock.

This study provided preliminary data showing the efficacy of injection therapy with peanut extract. A follow-up study recruited 12 patients who had immediate hypersensitivity to ingestion of peanuts [21]. Six subjects were treated with injections of peanut extract, in whom a maintenance level of tolerance was first achieved by a rush protocol and then maintained with weekly injections for at least 1 year. The other six were untreated control subjects. All patients underwent DBPCFC to peanut initially, after approximately 6 weeks, and after 1 year. All treated patients achieved the maintenance dose of 0.5 mL of 1:100 wt/vol peanut extract with the rush injection protocol. All experienced increased tolerance to DBPCFC and decreased sensitivity on titrated SPT with peanut extract, whereas the threshold to oral peanut challenge and cutaneous reactivity to peanut extract were unchanged in the untreated control subjects.

Systemic reactions were common in the treated group both during rush immunotherapy and with maintenance injections (39%). Only three patients remained tolerant of the full maintenance dose. The increased tolerance to oral peanut challenge was maintained in the three subjects treated with full maintenance doses, but the patients who required dose reduction because of systemic reactions experienced partial (n = 2) or complete (n = 1) loss of protection. In addition, no long-term follow-up data evaluated the persistence of protection after peanut immunotherapy discontinuation. Nevertheless, this pivotal clinical study showed that food allergen could be successfully used to induce oral tolerance in subjects who have food allergies if safety was improved. The authors concluded that modified peanut extract of decreased allergenicity was needed for future clinical applications.

Birch pollen immunotherapy for pollen–food allergy syndrome (oral allergy syndrome)

Cross-reactivity between birch tree pollen and allergens in raw apple is the basis for an approach that uses subcutaneous birch tree pollen immunotherapy to treat oral allergy to apple. Respiratory sensitization to pollen allergens (eg, major birch allergen, Bet v 1) that cross-react with allergens in plant foods (eg, major apple allergen, Mal d 1) results in oropharyngeal symptoms triggered by the ingestion of raw fruits and vegetables [22]. A prospective, nonrandomized, nonblinded clinical trial of birch pollen subcutaneous immunotherapy in 49 adults who had birch pollinosis and oral symptoms provoked by apple was recently reported [23]. Subjects underwent birch immunotherapy for 12, 24, or 36 months. After undergoing immunotherapy, 41 patients (84%) compared with no (0%) controls (birch-allergic adults who underwent no immunotherapy) reported a significant reduction (50%–95%) or total clearance (100%) of apple allergy symptoms ($P<.001$).

Birch immunotherapy also induced a marked reduction in skin reactivity against fresh apple in 43 patients (88%). The effect of immunotherapy was inversely related with baseline skin reactivity. In contrast, baseline birch pollen–specific or apple-specific IgE antibody levels did not correlate with immunotherapy effectiveness on apple allergy. No control subject reported a reduction in the severity of apple allergy or showed a decrease in skin reactivity at follow-up ($P < .001$). Immunotherapy with birch pollen extracts effectively reduced clinical apple sensitivity and skin reactivity in most cases after only 1 year of treatment.

These effects were not paralleled by a similar reduction in apple-specific IgE. In a follow-up study, the duration of the effect of birch immunotherapy was evaluated in 30 patients who had birch pollen allergy who experienced resolution of apple allergy and loss of skin-test reactivity to fresh apple [24]. Symptoms and skin-test reactivity were compared at the end of the immunotherapy course and 30 months after immunotherapy was stopped. More than 50% of patients were still able to tolerate eating apple at the 30-month follow-up visit, although most showed evidence of resensitization to apple on SPT. Both studies were criticized for lack of randomized design and objective evaluation of the severity of apple allergy using DBPCFC. However, despite limitations, these studies provided evidence that birch pollen immunotherapy may provide a long-lasting improvement in apple allergy in a subset of birch allergic individuals who have oral allergy to apple. Subsequent clinical trials, in which oral allergy to apple was diagnosed with DBPCFC, confirmed the beneficial effect of birch immunotherapy on oral tolerance to apple in some patients [25,26]. Asero [27] speculated that some patients who have oral allergy syndrome may need immunotherapy doses higher than typically needed to produce improvement in birch pollen rhinitis. He also pointed out that most significant effects on oral allergy syndrome were observed in the studies that included adults monosensitized to birch tree pollen and not to other pollens.

Oral desensitization in food allergy

Oral desensitization to food or, as proposed by Niggemann and colleagues [28], specific oral tolerance induction (SOTI) is generating increasing interest as a potential approach to treating food allergy [29]. The rationale for using the oral route is that oral ingestion of a food antigen results preferentially in the active nonresponse of the immune system toward that antigen. Animal studies suggest that high-dose feeding of an antigen results in anergy or deletion of the antigen-specific T lymphocytes, whereas intermittent feedings with small doses will more likely cause activation of the regulatory T cells and mediators [30]. Although some researchers postulate that food allergy results from the failure to develop, or a breech in, oral tolerance, direct evidence in humans has not been established.

With allergy to cow's milk, peanut, or egg, experts have assumed that the major route of sensitization is through the gastrointestinal tract because these proteins are resistant to proteolytic enzymes and low gastric pH [2]. In contrast, sensitization to proteins in raw fruits and vegetables that are highly cross-reactive with pollen allergens predominantly occurs through the respiratory tract and is primarily directed to inhaled pollen with subsequent reactivity to ingested cross-reactive food [31]. However, experimental murine models show that epicutaneous sensitization to food allergens preferentially induces Th 2 responses and results in allergic responses to inhaled and ingested food proteins [32–34].

In mice, oral tolerance induction is highly dose-dependent and differs for the allergenic proteins of peanut and egg ovalbumin [35]. Tolerance to peanut requires a significantly higher oral dose than does tolerance to ovalbumin. Low doses of peanut are more likely to induce oral sensitization and increase production of interleukin (IL)-4 and specific IgE on challenge. Retrospective epidemiologic data from the United Kingdom collected as maternal recall and subject to recall bias suggest that application of creams containing peanut oil is a risk factor for the development of peanut allergy in infants, especially in the setting of atopic dermatitis and impaired skin barrier [36]. In addition, up to 50% of children who have peanut and egg allergy experience their initial food allergic reaction to the first known ingestion of these foods, suggesting that prior exposures occurred either through unknown ingestion, such as resulting from cross-contamination of trace amounts from shared equipment, through transmission in breast milk, or potentially through an alternative route, such as skin or respiratory tract [37]. Because approximately 90% of children who have food allergy have atopic dermatitis and at least 40% to 50% of young children who have persistent moderate-to-severe atopic dermatitis have food allergy, epicutaneous sensitization to the common food allergens through impaired skin barrier may represent an important underappreciated route and provide the rationale for trials of oral tolerance induction to these foods.

Current evidence supporting oral desensitization is limited to nonrandomized clinical trials and case reports with little insight into the immunomodulatory effects of oral food desensitization (Table 1) [38–47]. In addition, because of methodology issues, the actual effects of oral desensitization versus the natural resolution of allergy to foods such as cow's milk and egg that are typically outgrown by most children is difficult to appreciate. Nevertheless, in many patients, tolerance to food seems to be achieved and maintained for up to 6 months if the food is ingested regularly [46,47]. However, in some patients who reach maintenance dose, allergic symptoms redevelop if the food is not ingested regularly, highlighting a concern as to whether oral desensitization is capable of inducing permanent tolerance [29].

In a subset of individuals, the full maintenance dose cannot be achieved because of adverse reactions, but the patients benefit from increased threshold dose of food. Patients are protected from reactions to trace amounts, and benefit from increased safety, comfort, and nutritional value when they continue to ingest the food on daily basis to guarantee maintenance of desensitization state [47]. Compared with subcutaneous allergen immunotherapy, the concept of oral immunomodulation and tolerance induction for therapy of food allergy is undeniably appealing, especially considering the low rate of serious adverse reactions and the comfort of home-administration. However, rigorous clinical trials are necessary to fully evaluate the role of oral desensitization in the definitive treatment of food allergy. Finally, mechanistic studies are needed to understand the immunologic changes induced by oral desensitization.

Sublingual immunotherapy with food extract

Another approach to food therapy is sublingual immunotherapy with food extracts. A recent randomized, double-blind, placebo-controlled trial evaluated sublingual immunotherapy for treating hazelnut allergy using commercial hazelnut extract [48]. Adult subjects who had hazelnut allergy confirmed with DBPCFC were randomly assigned to two treatment groups: hazelnut immunotherapy [11] or placebo [1]. Patients kept the immunotherapy solution in the mouth for at least 3 minutes and then discharged it. According to a rush schedule, all patients undergoing hazelnut immunotherapy reached the planned maximum dose in 4 days under physician supervision in the hospital, followed by home administration of a daily maintenance dose of five drops of the most potent extract over 5 months (November–March). The maintenance daily dose contained 188.2 μg of Cor a 1 and 121.9 μg of Cor a 8, major hazelnut allergens. Systemic reactions were observed in 0.2% of the total doses administered, were limited to the rush build-up phase, and were treated with oral antihistamines. Mean threshold dose of ingested hazelnut for objective symptoms increased from 2.3 g to 11.6 g ($P = .02$; active group) versus 3.5 g to 4.1 g ($P =$ not significant; placebo) at follow-up evaluation. Almost 50% of patients who underwent active treatment reached the highest dose (20 g) of hazelnut during follow-up DBPCFC compared with 9% in the placebo group. Levels of serum hazelnut-specific IgG_4 antibody and total serum IL-10 increased only in the active group, but no differences were seen in hazelnut-specific IgE antibody levels pre- and postimmunotherapy.

These preliminary data are encouraging, especially in terms of safety, but more studies are needed to determine optimal duration of immunotherapy and persistence of protective effect when immunotherapy is discontinued. In addition, immunotherapy trials with different food allergens and in different patient populations (eg, children versus adults and subjects who have well-defined anaphylactic reactivity to foods) must be conducted before the role of sublingual immunotherapy in treating food allergy can be determined.

Recombinant food proteins

In the past decade, tremendous progress was accomplished in identifying the relevant food proteins. Major food allergens, such as those in cow's milk, egg white, soybean, wheat, peanut, tree nuts, seeds, fish, and shellfish were characterized by their structure and function. Proteins cross-reactive

Table 1
Summary of current experience with oral food desensitization for IgE-mediated food allergy

Study	Foods	Subjects	Starting dose	Time to maintenance	Success rate[a]	Comments
Patriarca et al., 1984 [38] Open clinical trial	CM (8)	N = 19 Age: 5–55 years	10 drops of CM in 10 mL of water; 4 drops/d	100 mL of undiluted CM per day in 104 days	5/8	Side effects in 11/19 patients: urticaria, pruritus, emesis, angioedema, abdominal pain, rhinitis, dyspnea; patients followed up for 3–12 months; subject who had orange allergy reported resolution of allergy to plums and peaches; no insight into mechanism of desensitization
	Egg (8)		10 drops of beaten egg in 100 mL of water, 4 drops/d	120 drops of pure beaten egg per day in 90 days	6/8	
	Fish (2)		10 mL of mixed fish commercial extract (eel, sardine, codfish, anchovy) in 90 mL of water, 4 drops/d	200 g of cooked fish/day in 120 days	2/2	
	Orange (1)		Unspecified	3 months	1/1	
Patriarca et al., 1998 [39] Clinical trial	CM (6) Egg (5) Fish (2) Apple (1)	N = 14 Age: 4–14 years	Modification of previously published protocol [38]	Modification of previously published protocol [38]	12/14	All children who achieved maintenance continued to tolerate the foods at least 2–3 times per week for 3–6 years 10/14 patients experienced side effects during treatment
Bauer et al., 1999 [40]	CM	N = 1 Age 12 years	1 mL/d of 0.01% milk diluted in water	Rush protocol: dose doubled every other hour; final dose 200 mL of undiluted milk achieved in 5 days	1/1	Patient tolerated cow's milk daily for at least 6 months of follow-up

Nucera et al., 2000 [41]	Cow's milk	N = 1 Age 6 years	10 drops of milk in 10 mL of water; 4 drops per day	100 mL of undiluted cow's milk per day in 104 days	1/1	Child able to ingest CM and dairy products after 6 months; after 7 months; SPT to BLG, ALA, and CS became negative; IgE to milk proteins decreased significantly, whereas milk-IgG and IgA increased; PBMC stimulated with BLG produced significantly less IL-4 at 18 months than at baseline
Rueff et al., 2001 [42]	Celery	N = 1 Age: 49 years	0.1 mL of a commercial natural celery juice five times a day	5 mL five times daily for 3 months	1/1	At 3 months, patient tolerated 10 g of raw celery but developed flushing to 20 g; continued to ingest 25 mL per day of raw celery juice for 3 years
Patriarca et al., 2003 [46] Clinical trial	CM (29) Egg (15) Fish (11) Orange (2); and other[b]	N = 59 Age: 3–55 years	Modification of previously published protocol [38]	Modification of previously published protocol [38]	45/54 (83.3%)	51% of patients experienced urticaria, emesis, diarrhea, or abdominal pain; in 9 patients (16.7%), protocol was stopped because of side effects; no differences between children and adults; SPT became negative after 18 months in 78%; food-IgE decreased and food-IgG4 increased after 18 months
Meglio et al., 2004 [47]	CM	N = 21 Age: 5–10 years	1 drop of CM diluted 1:25 in water	200 mL undiluted CM per day over 180 days	15/21 (71.4%)	3/21 reacted to minimal dose of diluted CM; 3/21 tolerated only 40–80 CM per day; 15/21 tolerated 200 mL CM per day for 6 months; Side effect rate 13/21; SPT to BLG and CS significantly decreased at 6 months ($P<.001$), CM-IgE levels not significantly different

(*continued on next page*)

Table 1 (*continued*)

Study	Foods	Subjects	Starting dose	Time to maintenance	Success rate[a]	Comments
Rolinck-Werninghaus et al., 2005 [29]	CM (1) Egg (2)	N = 3 Age: 4–12 years	0.0006 mL of CM per day; 0.01 mg egg per day at home	100 mL CM per day over 37 weeks, 2.5 g egg per day (1/2 egg) over 41–52 weeks	3/3	All patients had acute symptoms to food re-exposure after discontinuation of food for 2–14 days; the only study to rechallenge patients to food after a period of avoidance while on maintenance
Patriarca et al., 2006 [43]	Peanut	N = 1	5.6 mg peanut per day on day 1	40 g peanut per day over 7 days in the hospital	1/1	SPT to peanut became negative at 6 months, no significant changes in peanut-IgE (baseline: 2.1, 6 months: 1.5) or peanut-IgG
Pons et al., 2006 [44]	Egg white	N = 3	Not specified	Rush immunotherapy on day 1 in the hospital, then build-up over several months	3/3	Percentage of egg-specific CD4+CD23high T cells increased starting between 3 and 6 months, in parallel with production of IL-10 by egg white–stimulated PBMC
Buchanan et al., 2006 [45]	Peanut	N = 7 Mean age 4.4 years	Not specified	Rush phase and dose escalation in the hospital, maintenance at home	7/7 at 6 months	During rush phase 4/7 required oral antihistamine; at 6 months a mean 2.3-fold increase in peanut-IgG and mean change in peanut-IgE of 0.9-fold occurred

Abbreviations: ALA, alpha-lactalbumin; BLG, beta-lactoglobulin; CM, cow's milk; CS, casein; PBMC, peripheral blood mononuclear cells; SPT, skin prick test.

[a] Success rate defined as regular ingestion of the tested food for at least 6 months.

[b] One of each: apple, peach, lettuce, orange, beans, and corn.

with birch tree pollen found in foods of plant origin (eg, fruits, vegetables, legumes, and tree nuts) responsible for oral allergy syndrome were extensively studied [31]. Severity of peanut allergy was correlated with the diversity of epitopes recognized on the major peanut allergens, Ara h 1, Ara h 2, and Ara h 3, by B cells [49–51]. Individuals allergic to cow's milk, egg, and peanut who had no IgE antibodies against certain sequential epitopes of the major allergens were found to be more likely to achieve tolerance than subjects whose IgE antibodies were directed against those epitopes [52–55].

Identification of the most relevant food allergens was followed by generation of recombinant proteins [56]. To date, a significant number of recombinant food allergens have been synthesized, including major peanut allergens (Ara h 1, 2, and 3); major allergens from English walnut (Jug r 1), hazelnut (Cor a 1.04), and cashew (Ana o 1); tropomyosins from crab, lobster, shrimp, and snail; parvalbumins from salmon, carp, and codfish; lipid transfer proteins from carrot, bell pepper, tomato, wheat, and cherry; birch Bet v 1 cross-reactive major allergens from carrot, apple, and celery; soybean glycinin; and egg white ovomucoid. Most recombinant food proteins were evaluated in regard to their ability to bind specific IgE antibody from allergic patients' sera, and some were used for skin prick testing [51,57,58]. The availability of pure recombinant allergens should enable customization of diagnostic tests and result in more precise testing for individuals who have food allergies. It should also allow for improved safety of testing procedures by eliminating contaminations and undeclared allergens in wild-type allergen extracts [59].

Animal models of food hypersensitivity

Because of ethical concerns about serious side effects of food immunotherapy, animal models were crucial in evaluating efficacy and safety of experimental therapies. Li and colleagues [60,61] developed well-characterized murine models of IgE-mediated cow's milk and peanut hypersensitivity in which subjects were sensitized orally and developed anaphylaxis after oral feeding. In the peanut model, C3H/HeJ mice were sensitized orally with freshly ground whole peanut and cholera toxin as adjuvant and challenged orally 3 and 5 weeks later with crude peanut extract [61]. Peanut-specific IgE was induced through oral peanut sensitization, and hypersensitivity reactions were provoked by feeding peanut to sensitized mice. The symptoms were similar to those seen in human subjects (Fig. 2). Ara h 1– and Ara h 2–specific IgE antibodies were present in the sera of mice with peanut allergy. Furthermore, these Ara h 2–specific IgE antibodies bound the same Ara h 2 isoforms and major allergenic epitopes as antibodies in the sera of humans who had peanut allergy. Splenocytes from mice with peanut allergy exhibited proliferative responses to Ara h 1 and Ara h 2. This murine model of peanut allergy mimics the clinical and immunologic characteristics

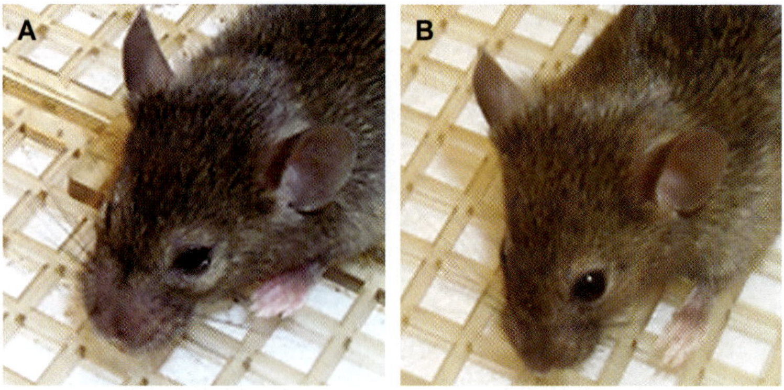

Fig. 2. Murine model of peanut anaphylaxis. (*A*) Peanut allergic–mouse showing edema of the snout, eye, and paws, and pilar erecti after oral peanut challenge (score 3) (*B*) Non–peanut allergic mouse asymptomatic on feeding with peanut (score 0). C3H/HeJ mice were sensitized intragastrically with PN and cholera toxin on days 0, 7, and 14. At week 3, mice were challenged with 10 mg of crude peanut extract intragastrically. Symptoms were scored using a 0- to 5-point scale, with 0 indicating no signs of reaction and 5 indicating death. (*Reprinted from* Li XM, Srivastava K, Grishin A, et al. Persistent protective effect of heat-killed Escherichia coli producing "engineered," recombinant peanut proteins in a murine model of peanut allergy. J Allergy Clin Immunol 2003;112(1):159–67; with permission. Copyright © 2003, American Academy of Allergy, Asthma, and Immunology.)

of peanut allergy in humans and has been used subsequently in many studies.

Immunotherapeutic approaches based on recombinant food proteins

An early study found that the intramuscular immunization of naïve AKR/J (H-2^K) and C3H/HeJ (H-2^K) mice with plasmid DNA encoding Ara h 2 before intraperitoneal peanut sensitization had some protective effects in AKR/J mice, but induced anaphylactic reactions in peanut-sensitized C3H/HeJ mice after peanut challenge [62]. Li and colleagues [62] also found no reduction in peanut–IgE antibody levels and more severe anaphylactic symptoms after oral challenge in peanut-allergic mice that were treated with pDNA-expressing Ara H 2. However, in another study, oral chitosan–embedded Ara h 2 had a protective effect in preventing sensitization in AKR mice [63]. These data indicate that pDNA-based immunotherapy may not be effective in reversing established IgE-mediated hypersensitivity.

Conjugated allergen administration with synthetic immunostimulatory oligodeoxynucleotides containing unmethylated CpG motifs (ISS) was more effective than a mixture of antigen and ISS in suppressing allergic airway responses, probably because of the enhanced dendritic cell uptake of ISS-allergen. Srivastava and colleagues [64] explored the concept of ISS potentiation of Th 1 responses to food allergens through immunizing

C3H/HeJ mice intradermally with either ISS-linked Ara h 2, or ISS-linked Amb a 1 as a control. Four weeks after immunization, mice were intragastrically sensitized with peanut and challenged with Ara h 2 5 weeks later. Mice treated with ISS–Ara h 2 did not develop symptoms and had significantly lower plasma histamine levels after oral challenge compared with those treated with ISS–Amb a 1.

Nguyen and colleagues [65] found that intradermal immunization with a mixture of ISS and β-gal, but not with ISS alone or β-gal alone, provided protection against fatal anaphylaxis induced by intraperitoneal β-gal sensitization and challenge that was associated with an increase in IgG2a/interferon (IFN)-γ and a reduction in IgE/IL-4 and IL-5. This effect was comparable to immunization with the pDNA-encoding β-gal. These results suggest that antigen–ISS immunization may have a prophylactic effect against allergy. However, the ability to reverse established food allergy remains to be determined.

Recombinant engineered food proteins

Immunotherapy with native peanut was found to have an unacceptably high rate of adverse reactions to immunotherapy injections, but the concept of using immunomodulation with peanut protein to increase oral tolerance to peanut was confirmed [20,21]. Subsequent studies concentrated on generating hypoallergenic recombinant peanut proteins that lost the ability to interact with IgE antibodies directed against native peanut but retained the ability to interact with T cells. These engineered recombinant peanut proteins were expected not to activate mast cells and thus ensure an improved safety profile.

In the initial study, peanut major allergen Ara h 1 was cloned and characterized as a member of the vicillin storage protein family [66]. RNA isolated from peanut species (Florunner) was used to construct an expression library through western blot analysis for screening with serum IgE from patients who had peanut allergy. Several clones were selected with intense binding to sera of patients who had peanut allergy. When incubated with these sera, allergens from 94% of patients that bound to wild-type Ara h 1 also bound to recombinant Ara h 1.

Subsequently, two additional major peanut allergens were cloned and characterized: Ara h 2 and Ara h 3 [67–69]. The IgE-binding epitopes of these allergens have been determined. Amino acids critical to each epitope were identified, and site-directed mutagenesis of the allergen cDNA clones was used to produce engineered recombinant allergens. Engineered recombinant peanut allergens were then analyzed through immunoblotting with peanut-allergic patients' sera [70]. Fifty-seven patients were tested for IgE binding to Ara h 1, 52 patients for Ara h 2, and 52 patients for Ara h 3. IgE binding to engineered recombinant allergens ranged from 5.4% to 125% of wild-type Ara h 1, 0% to 99.8% of wild-type Ara h 2, and 19.3% to 141%

of wild-type Ara h 3. Peripheral blood mononuclear cells (PBMC) from subjects who had peanut allergy were incubated with engineered recombinant peanut allergens and proliferation was assessed through the incorporation of radioactive thymidine into the DNA of dividing cells. PBMCs from 12 individuals who had peanut allergy were tested for each wild-type and engineered recombinant allergen. The average stimulation index produced by the engineered recombinant allergens in comparison to its wild-type counterpart was 72% for Ara h 1, 104% for Ara h 2, and 72% for Ara h 3.

Subsequently, wild-type Ara h 2 and engineered recombinant Ara h 2 were compared in their ability to interact with T cells, bind IgE, and release mediators from passively sensitized RBL-2H3 cell line. Multiple T-cell epitopes were identified on Ara h 2. Amino acid regions of Ara h 2, 11–35, 86–125, and 121–155 contained most peptides that interact with T cells from patients who had peanut allergy. Wild-type and engineered recombinant Ara h 2 stimulated proliferation of T cells from patients who had peanut allergy to similar levels. In contrast, engineered recombinant Ara h 2 greatly reduced IgE-binding capacity and released significantly lower amounts of β-hexosaminidase, a marker of IgE-mediated RBL-2H3 degranulation, compared with the wild-type allergen [71]. These studies showed that the engineered recombinant peanut allergens retained the ability to interact with T cells while they lost the ability to interact with IgE antibodies directed against native peanut proteins, supporting their use in trials of peanut immunotherapy.

Recombinant major apple allergen (rMal d 1) with five-point mutations introduced by site-directed mutagenesis was recently evaluated in 14 adults who had birch tree pollen and apple allergy [58]. IgE reactivity to mutated rMal d 1 was twofold lower than that of the wild-type molecule (95% CI; 1.7–2.4). Radioallergosorbent test (RAST) inhibition showed a 7.8-fold decrease in IgE-binding capacity (95% CI; 3.0–12.6). The biologic activity of mutant rMal d 1 assessed with SPT and basophil histamine release decreased 10- to 200-fold. In addition, DBPCFC in two subjects confirmed lower allergenicity of mutant rMal d 1 compared with wild-type rMal d 1, as measured by increased threshold dose, inducing symptoms, and maximum severity of reaction at the peak dose. This study was the first to show hypoallergenicity of engineered recombinant food allergen through an oral food challenge. These results are encouraging, but must be interpreted cautiously, because point mutations may result in formation of new allergenic epitopes and paradoxically increase allergenicity of mutated allergens for some patients [70].

Engineered recombinant peanut immunotherapy

In vivo efficacy of the engineered recombinant peanut proteins was tested in the murine model of peanut anaphylaxis [72]. Mice were sensitized to whole peanut and then desensitized through intranasal administration of engineered recombinant Ara h 2 (three doses per week for 4 weeks).

Desensitization with the engineered recombinant Ara h 2 protein suppressed synthesis of Ara h 2–IgE and resulted in significantly decreased symptoms on oral peanut challenge compared with a control group treated with wild-type Ara h 2.

Engineered recombinant peanut proteins mixed with bacterial adjuvants immunotherapy

Bacteria are potent stimulants of Th 1 immune responses and increase IFN-γ production. Heat-killed *Listeria monocytogenes* (HKLM) was shown to reverse established allergic airway hyperreactivity in mice [73]. In a dog model, a single subcutaneous treatment with a mixture of HKLM, milk, and wheat significantly reduced immediate skin test reactions and prevented anaphylactic symptoms on oral food challenge [74]. Li and colleagues [75] tested the efficacy of a mixture of HKLM and modified peanut proteins (Ara h 1, Ara h 2, and Ara h 3). Peanut-allergic C3H/HeJ mice were treated 10 weeks after sensitization with a mixture of the three major peanut allergens and HKLM (modified [m]Ara h 1–3 plus HKLM) administered subcutaneously. All mice in the sham-treated groups exhibited anaphylactic symptoms with a median symptom score of 3, whereas only 31% of mice in the mAra h 1–3 plus HKLM group developed mild anaphylaxis, with a low median symptom score of 0.5 on a scale of 0 to 5. Changes in core body temperature, bronchial constriction, plasma histamine, and peanut-specific IgE levels were all significantly reduced. This protective effect was markedly more potent than in the group treated with mAra h 1–3 protein

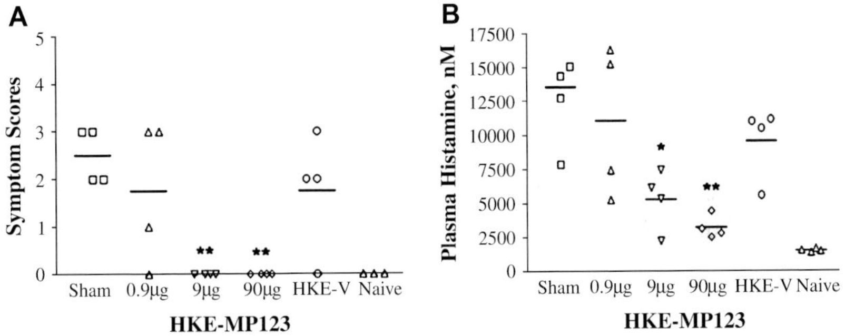

Fig. 3. Persistent protection against peanut-induced anaphylactic reactions by HKE-MP123. Mice were challenged at 10 weeks after the last HKE-MP123 treatment. (*A*) Anaphylactic symptom scores were determined 30 minutes after challenge. Each point indicates an individual mouse. Bars indicate the median of four mice in each group. (*B*) Histamine plasma levels were measured in blood samples obtained 30 to 40 minutes after the challenge. Data are means +SEM for each group of four mice. **P*<.05, and ***P*<.01 versus sham. (*Reprinted from* Li XM, Srivastava K, Grishin A, et al. Persistent protective effect of heat-killed *Escherichia coli* producing "engineered," recombinant peanut proteins in a murine model of peanut allergy. J Allergy Clin Immunol 2003;112(1):159–67; with permission. Copyright © 2003, American Academy of Allergy, Asthma, and Immunology.)

Table 2
Comparison of native, recombinant, and engineered recombinant allergen immunotherapy for food allergy

Therapy	Mechanism of action	Effects	Comments
Conventional peanut IT	Altered T-cell responses, up-regulation of suppressor cells in allergen IT	Increased oral peanut tolerance	Subcutaneous injections of gradually increasing doses of allergen, unacceptably high rate of serious adverse events
Birch pollen IT for oral allergy to apple	Marked reduction in skin test to raw apple; IT inversely correlated with baseline skin test but not with serum apple or birch-IgE	Significant reduction or total resolution of oral allergy to raw Golden Delicious apple in a subset of patients undergoing IT for at least 12 months	Clinical effect lasting for up to 30 months after discontinuation in >50% of patients
Oral desensitization	Presumed oral tolerance induction; decreased skin test reactivity, increased serum food-IgG/IgG4, no change in food-IgE, increased food-specific CD4+CD23 high T cells, increased IL-10 on food antigen stimulation	Tolerance to regular servings of food in most subjects (70%–80%) maintained as long as food ingested on regular basis for up to 6 months; in a subset increased threshold dose for clinical reactions	Up to 50% experience systemic side effects; some patients require uninterrupted ingestion of food to maintain desensitized tolerant state; rigorous clinical trials necessary to determine safety and efficacy
Sublingual IT with hazelnut extract	Presumed oral tolerance induction; increased serum hazelnut-IgG4 and total IL-10 level, no change in hazelnut-IgE	Increased oral hazelnut tolerance	Systemic reactions in only 0.2% of doses during build-up phase, treated with oral antihistamines; rigorous clinical trials necessary to determine safety and efficacy

Plasmid DNA–based IT	Induces prolonged humoral and cellular responses because of CpG motifs in the DNA backbone	Protection against peanut anaphylaxis in sensitized AKR/J mice, but induction of anaphylaxis in C3H/HeJ ($H-2^K$) mice; no effect on peanut-IgE antibody levels	Serious concerns regarding safety in view of strain-dependent effects in mice, concern for excessive Th 1 stimulation and autoimmunity
Immunostimulatory sequences (ISS-ODN)	Potent stimulation of Th 1 through activation of antigen-presenting cells, natural killer cells, and B cells; increased Th 1 cytokines	Protection against peanut sensitization in mice	Not shown to reverse established peanut allergy, concern for excessive Th 1 stimulation, and potential for autoimmunity
Engineered recombinant peanut IT	Binding to mast cells eliminated, T-cell responses comparable to native peanut allergens	Protection against peanut anaphylaxis in mice	Improved safety profile compared with conventional IT, requires identification of IgE binding sites
Heat-killed bacteria mixed with or expressing engineered recombinant peanut proteins	Potentiation of Th 1 and T-regulatory cytokine responses	Protection against peanut anaphylaxis in mice, lasting up to 10 weeks after treatment	Concern for toxicity of bacterial adjuvants, excessive Th 1 stimulation, and potential for autoimmunity; heat-killed *Escherichia coli* expressing modified peanut allergens administered rectally viewed as the safest approach for future human studies

Abbreviation: IT, immunotherapy.

alone. HKLM alone showed no protective effect. Reduced IL-5 and IL-13 and increased IFN-γ levels were observed only in peanut-stimulated splenocyte cultures from mice treated with mAra h 1–3 plus HKLM. These results showed that immunotherapy with modified peanut proteins and HKLM was effective in treating peanut allergy in this model, and might be a potential treatment approach.

Because of safety concerns about using potentially pathogenic bacteria in humans, a nonpathogenic strain of *Escherichia coli* was selected as a bacterial adjuvant. Subsequent studies investigated heat-killed *E coli* (HKE) expressing modified peanut proteins administered subcutaneously and found that lower doses were required for desensitization [76]. However, considering potential complications resulting from subcutaneous administration in humans, further studies focused on the vaccine administered per rectum. Because nonpathogenic *E coli* bacteria reside in the colon, experts assumed that rectal delivery would provide superior safety regarding possible infectious complications and severe adverse reactions. In addition, the rectal route is noninvasive and could be safely used in young children who would probably be the target for this vaccine.

The long-term immunomodulatory effect of HKE producing mutated Ara h 1, 2, and 3 (HKE–MP123) administered rectally was investigated in a murine model of peanut anaphylaxis [77]. Peanut-allergic C3H/HeJ mice received 0.9 μg (low-dose), 9 μg (medium-dose), or 90 μg (high-dose) HKE-MP123 administered rectally; HKE-containing vector (HKE-V) alone; or vehicle alone (sham) weekly for 3 weeks. Mice were challenged 2 weeks later. Second and third challenges were performed at 4-week intervals. After the first challenge, all three groups treated with HKE-MP123 and HKE-V showed reduced symptom scores ($P<.01$, .01, .05, and .05, respectively) compared with the sham-treated group. Only the medium- and high-dose HKE-MP123–treated mice remained protected for up to 10 weeks after treatment, accompanied by a significant reduction of plasma histamine levels compared with sham-treated mice ($P<.05$ and .01, respectively) (Fig. 3). IgE levels were significantly lower in all HKE-MP123–treated groups ($P<.001$), and were most reduced in the high-dose HKE-MP123–treated group at each challenge. In vitro IL-4, IL-13, IL-5, and IL-10 production by peanut-stimulated splenocytes of mice treated with high-dose HKE-MP123 were significantly decreased ($P<.01$, .001, .001, and .001, respectively), and IFN-γ and transforming growth factor β production were significantly increased ($P<.001$ and .01, respectively) compared with sham-treated mice at the last challenge. Treatment with rectal HKE-MP123 can induce long-term down-regulation of peanut hypersensitivity, which might be secondary to decreased antigen-specific Th 2 and increased Th 1 and T-regulatory cytokine production. The rectal vaccine is currently being standardized in preparation for a phase I human clinical trial. Table 2 compares experience with native, recombinant, and engineered recombinant allergen immunotherapy for food allergy.

Non–allergen-specific approaches to food allergy treatment

In addition to research focusing on immunotherapy with native and engineered recombinant food proteins, alternative approaches to food allergy therapy have been investigated, including monoclonal anti-IgE therapy, Chinese herbs, and cytokine therapy [78–82].

Summary

Food allergy is a serious medical problem without definitive treatment at this time. Intense research focuses on severe peanut allergy. Recombinant peanut major allergens engineered to lose IgE-binding capacity mixed with *E coli* showed great promise in a murine model of peanut anaphylaxis. Rectal vaccine containing *E coli* expressing engineered recombinant major peanut allergens Ara h 1, 2, and 3 is in preparation for first human clinical trials. Oral desensitization and sublingual immunotherapy with food extracts represent another approach that is being actively explored. Novel therapies must be evaluated carefully regarding safety and long-lasting effect on oral food tolerance before being applied in clinical practice. Diversity of approaches and promising preliminary results bring hope for patients who have food allergy.

References

[1] Sicherer SH, Sampson HA. Food allergy. J Allergy Clin Immunol 2006;117(2 Suppl Mini-Primer):S470–5.
[2] Sampson HA. Food allergy. J Allergy Clin Immunol 2003;111(Suppl 2):S540–7.
[3] Yocum MW, Butterfield JH, Klein JS, et al. Epidemiology of anaphylaxis in Olmested County: a population-based study. J Allergy Clin Immunol 1999;104:452–6.
[4] Sicherer SH, Munoz-Furlong A, Burks AW, et al. Prevalence of peanut and tree nut allergy in the US determined by a random digit dial telephone survey. J Allergy Clin Immunol 1999; 103(4):559–62.
[5] Sicherer SH, Munoz-Furlong A, Sampson HA. Prevalence of peanut and tree nut allergy in the United States determined by means of a random digit dial telephone survey: a 5-year follow-up study. J Allergy Clin Immunol 2003;112(6):1203–7.
[6] Sicherer SA, Munoz-Furlong A, Sampson HA. Prevalence of seafood allergy in the United States determined by a random telephone survey. J Allergy Clin Immunol 2004;114(1):159–65.
[7] Sicherer SH. Clinical implications of cross-reactive food allergens. J Allergy Clin Immunol 2001;108(6):881–90.
[8] Skolnick HS, Conover-Walker MK, Koerner CB, et al. The natural history of peanut allergy. J Allergy Clin Immunol 2001;107(2):367–74.
[9] Wood RA. The natural history of food allergy. Pediatrics 2003;111(6 Pt 3):1631–7.
[10] Fleischer DM, Conover-Walker MK, Matsui EC, et al. The natural history of tree nut allergy. J Allergy Clin Immunol 2005;116(5):1087–93.
[11] Bock SA, Sampson HA, Atkins FM, et al. Double-blind, placebo-controlled food challenge (DBPCFC) as an office procedure: a manual. J Allergy Clin Immunol 1988;82:986–97.
[12] Sampson HA, Ho DG. Relationship between food-specific IgE concentrations and the risk of positive food challenges in children and adolescents. J Allergy Clin Immunol 1997;444–51.

[13] Sampson HA. Utility of food-specific IgE concentrations in prediciting symptomatic food allergy. J Allergy Clin Immunol 2001;107:891–6.
[14] Bock SA, Atkins FM. The natural history of peanut allergy. J Allergy Clin Immunol 1989; 83(5):900–4.
[15] Grundy J, Matthews S, Bateman B, et al. Rising prevalence of allergy to peanut in children: data from 2 sequential cohorts. J Allergy Clin Immunol 2002;110(5):784–9.
[16] Kagan RS, Joseph L, Dufresne C, et al. Prevalence of peanut allergy in primary-school children in Montreal, Canada. J Allergy Clin Immunol 2003;112(6):1223–8.
[17] Bock SA, Munoz-Furlong A, Sampson HA. Fatalities due to anaphylactic reactions to foods. J Allergy Clin Immunol 2001;107(1):191–3.
[18] American Academy of Pediatrics. Committee on Nutrition. Hypoallergenic infant formulas. Pediatrics 2000;106(2):346–9.
[19] Nelson HS. Advances in upper airway diseases and allergen immunotherapy. J Allergy Clin Immunol 2006;117(5):1047–53.
[20] Oppenheimer JJ, Nelson HS, Bock SA, et al. Treatment of peanut allergy with rush immunotherapy. J Allergy Clin Immunol 1992;90(2):256–62.
[21] Nelson HS, Lahr J, Rule R, et al. Treatment of anaphylactic sensitivity to peanuts by immunotherapy with injections of aqueous peanut extract. J Allergy Clin Immunol 1997; 99(6 Pt 1):744–51.
[22] Valenta R, Kraft D. Type I allergic reactions to plant-derived food: a consequence of primary sensitization to pollen allergens. J Allergy Clin Immunol 1996;97:893–5.
[23] Asero R. Effects of birch pollen-specific immunotherapy on apple allergy in birch pollen-hypersensitive patients. Clin Exp Allergy 1998;28:1368–73.
[24] Asero R. How long does the effect of birch pollen injection SIT on apple allergy last? Allergy 2003;58(5):435–8.
[25] Bucher X, Pichler WJ, Dahinden CA, et al. Effect of tree pollen specific, subcutaneous immunotherapy on the oral allergy syndrome to apple and hazelnut. Allergy 2004;59(12): 1272–6.
[26] Bolhaar ST, Tiemessen MM, Zuidmeer L, et al. Efficacy of birch-pollen immunotherapy on cross-reactive food allergy confirmed by skin tests and double-blind food challenges. Clin Exp Allergy 2004;34(5):761–9.
[27] Asero R. Effects of birch pollen SIT on apple allergy: a matter of dosage? Allergy 2004; 59(12):1269–71.
[28] Niggemann B, Staden U, Rolinck-Werninghaus C, et al. Specific oral tolerance induction in food allergy. Allergy 2006;61(7):808–11.
[29] Rolinck-Werninghaus C, Staden U, Mehl A, et al. Specific oral tolerance induction with food in children: transient or persistent effect on food allergy? Allergy 2005;60(10):1320–2.
[30] Ko J, Mayer L. Oral tolerance: lessons on treatment of food allergy. Eur J Gastroenterol Hepatol 2005;17(12):1299–303.
[31] Vieths S, Scheurer S, Ballmer-Weber B. Current understanding of cross-reactivity of food allergens and pollen. Ann N Y Acad Sci 2002;964:47–68.
[32] Spergel JM, Mizoguchi E, Brewer JP, et al. Epicutaneous sensitization with protein antigen induces localized allergic dermatitis and hyperresponsiveness to methacholine after single exposure to aerosolized antigen in mice. J Clin Invest 1998;101(8): 1614–22.
[33] Hsieh KY, Tsai CC, Wu CH, et al. Epicutaneous exposure to protein antigen and food allergy. Clin Exp Allergy 2003;33(8):1067–75.
[34] Strid J, Hourihane J, Kimber I, et al. Epicutaneous exposure to peanut protein prevents oral tolerance and enhances allergic sensitization. Clin Exp Allergy 2005;35(6):757–66.
[35] Strid J, Thomson M, Hourihane J, et al. A novel model of sensitization and oral tolerance to peanut protein. Immunology 2004;113(3):293–303.
[36] Lack G, Fox D, Northstone K, et al. Factors associated with the development of peanut allergy in childhood. N Engl J Med 2003;348(11):977–85.

[37] Vadas P, Wai Y, Burks AW, et al. Detection of peanut allergens in breast milk of lactating women. JAMA 2001;285(13):1746–8.
[38] Patriarca C, Romano A, Venuti A, et al. Oral specific hyposensitization in the management of patients allergic to food. Allergol Immunopathol (Madr) 1984;12(4):275–81.
[39] Patriarca G, Schiavino D, Nucera E, et al. Food allergy in children: results of a standardized protocol for oral desensitization. Hepatogastroenterology 1998;45(19):52–8.
[40] Bauer A, Ekanayake MS, Wigger-Alberti W, et al. Oral rush desensitization to milk. Allergy 1999;54(8):894–5.
[41] Nucera E, Schiavino D, D'Ambrosio C, et al. Immunological aspects of oral desensitization in food allergy. Dig Dis Sci 2000;45(3):637–41.
[42] Rueff F, Eberlein-Konig B, Przybilla B. Oral hyposensitization with celery juice. Allergy 2001;56(1):82–3.
[43] Patriarca G, Nucera E, Pollastrini E, et al. Oral rush desensitization in peanut allergy: a case report. Dig Dis Sci 2006;51(3):471–3.
[44] Pons L, Buchanan AD, Steel PH, et al. CD4+CD25 high T regulatory cells in egg-allergic children undergoing oral desensitization. J Allergy Clin Immunol 2006;117(2):S42.
[45] Buchanan AD, Scurlock AM, Jone SM, et al. Oral desensitization and induction of tolerance in peanut-allergic children. J Allergy Clin Immunol 2006;117(2):S327.
[46] Patriarca G, Nucera E, Roncallo C, et al. Oral desensitizing treatment in food allergy: clinical and immunological results. Aliment Pharmacol Ther 2003;17(3):459–65.
[47] Meglio P, Bartone E, Plantamura M, et al. A protocol for oral desensitization in children with IgE-mediated cow's milk allergy. Allergy 2004;59(9):980–7.
[48] Enrique E, Pineda F, Malek T, et al. Sublingual immunotherapy for hazelnut food allergy: a randomized, double-blind, placebo-controlled study with a standardized hazelnut extract. J Allergy Clin Immunol 2005;116(5):1073–9.
[49] Shreffler WG, Lencer DA, Bardina L, et al. IgE and IgG4 epitope mapping by microarray immunoassay reveals the diversity of immune response to the peanut allergen, Ara h 2. J Allergy Clin Immunol 2005;116(4):893–9.
[50] Lewis SA, Grimshaw KE, Warner JO, et al. The promiscuity of immunoglobulin E binding to peanut allergens, as determined by Western blotting, correlates with the severity of clinical symptoms. Clin Exp Allergy 2005;35(6):767–73.
[51] Astier C, Morisset M, Roitel O, et al. Predictive value of skin prick tests using recombinant allergens for diagnosis of peanut allergy. J Allergy Clin Immunol 2006; 118(1):250–6.
[52] Beyer K, Ellman-Grunther L, Jarvinen KM, et al. Measurement of peptide-specific IgE as an additional tool in identifying patients with clinical reactivity to peanuts. J Allergy Clin Immunol 2003;112(1):202–7.
[53] Cooke SK, Sampson HA. Allergenic properties of ovomucoid in man. J Immunol 1997; 159(4):2026–32.
[54] Jarvinen KM, Chatchatee P, Bardina L, et al. IgE and IgG binding epitopes on alpha-lactalbumin and beta-lactoglobulin in cow's milk allergy. Int Arch Allergy Immunol 2001; 126(2):111–8.
[55] Jarvinen KM, Beyer K, Vila L, et al. B-cell epitopes as a screening instrument for persistent cow's milk allergy. J Allergy Clin Immunol 2002;110(2):293–7.
[56] Valenta R, Vrtala S, Laffer S, et al. Recombinant allergens. Allergy 1998;53(6):552–61.
[57] Reuter A, Lidholm J, Andersson K, et al. A critical assessment of allergen component-based in vitro diagnosis in cherry allergy across Europe. Clin Exp Allergy 2006;36(6): 815–23.
[58] Bolhaar ST, Zuidmeer L, Ma Y, et al. A mutant of the major apple allergen, Mal d 1, demonstrating hypo-allergenicity in the target organ by double-blind placebo-controlled food challenge. Clin Exp Allergy 2005;35(12):1638–44.
[59] Lidholm J, Ballmer-Weber BK, Mari A, et al. Component-resolved diagnostics in food allergy. Curr Opin Allergy Clin Immunol 2006;6(3):234–40.

[60] Li XM, Schofield BH, Huang CK, et al. A murine model of IgE-mediated cow's milk hypersensitivity. J Allergy Clin Immunol 1999;103(2 Pt 1):206–14.
[61] Li XM, Serebrisky D, Lee SY, et al. A murine model of peanut anaphylaxis: T- and B-cell responses to a major peanut allergen mimic human responses. J Allergy Clin Immunol 2000;106(1 Pt 1):150–8.
[62] Li X, Huang CK, Schofield BH, et al. Strain-dependent induction of allergic sensitization caused by peanut allergen DNA immunization in mice. J Immunol 1999;162(5):3045–52.
[63] Roy K, Mao HQ, Huang SK, et al. Oral gene delivery with chitosan–DNA nanoparticles generates immunologic protection in a murine model of peanut allergy. Nat Med 1999; 5(4):387–91.
[64] Srivastava K, Li XM, Bannon GA, et al. Investigation of the use of ISS-linked Ara h2 for the treatment of peanut-induced allergy [abstract]. J Allergy Clin Immunol 2001;107: S233.
[65] Nguyen MD, Cinman N, Yen J, et al. DNA-based vaccination for the treatment of food allergy. Allergy 2001;56(Suppl 67):127–30.
[66] Burks AW, Cockrell G, Stanley JS, et al. Recombinant peanut allergen Ara h I expression and IgE binding in patients with peanut hypersensitivity. J Clin Invest 1995;96(4): 1715–21.
[67] Eigenmann PA, Burks AW, Bannon GA, et al. Identification of unique peanut and soy allergens in sera adsorbed with cross-reacting antibodies. J Allergy Clin Immunol 1996; 98(5 Pt 1):969–78.
[68] Stanley JS, King N, Burks AW, et al. Identification and mutational analysis of the immunodominant IgE binding epitopes of the major peanut allergen Ara h 2. Arch Biochem Biophys 1997;342(2):244–53.
[69] Rabjohn P, Helm EM, Stanley JS, et al. Molecular cloning and epitope analysis of the peanut allergen Ara h 3. J Clin Invest 1999;103(4):535–42.
[70] Bannon GA, Cockrell G, Connaughton C, et al. Engineering, characterization and in vitro efficacy of the major peanut allergens for use in immunotherapy. Int Arch Allergy Immunol 2001;124(1–3):70–2.
[71] King N, Helm R, Stanley JS, et al. Allergenic characteristics of a modified peanut allergen. Mol Nutr Food Res 2005;49(10):963–71.
[72] Srivastava KD, Li XM, King N, et al. Immunotherapy with modified peanut allergens in a murine model of peanut allergy. J Allergy Clin Immunol 2002;109:S287.
[73] Yeung VP, Gieni RS, Umetsu DT, et al. Heat-killed *Listeria monocytogene* as an adjuvant converts established murine TH2-dominated immune responses into TH1-dominated responses. J Immunol 1998;161:4146–52.
[74] Frick OL, Bachanan BB, Delval G, et al. Allergen immunotherapy with heat-killed *Listeria monocytogenes* as adjuvant prevents allergic reactions in highly sensitized dogs [abstract]. J Allergy Clin Immunol 2001;107:S232.
[75] Li XM, Srivastava K, Huleatt JW, et al. Engineered recombinant peanut protein and heat-killed Listeria monocytogenes coadministration protects against peanut-induced anaphylaxis in a murine model. J Immunol 2003;170(6):3289–95.
[76] Stanley JS, Buzen F, Cockrell G, et al. Immunotherapy for peanut allergy using modified allergens and a bacterial adjuvant. J Allergy Clin Immunol 2002;109(1): S93.
[77] Li XM, Srivastava K, Grishin A, et al. Persistent protective effect of heat-killed Escherichia coli producing "engineered," recombinant peanut proteins in a murine model of peanut allergy. J Allergy Clin Immunol 2003;112(1):159–67.
[78] Leung DY, Sampson HA, Yunginger JW, et al. Effect of anti-IgE therapy in patients with peanut allergy. N Engl J Med 2003;348(11):986–93.
[79] Srivastava KD, Kattan JD, Zou ZM, et al. The Chinese herbal medicine formula FAHF-2 completely blocks anaphylactic reactions in a murine model of peanut allergy. J Allergy Clin Immunol 2005;115(1):171–8.

[80] Hsieh KY, Hsu CI, Lin JY, et al. Oral administration of an edible-mushroom-derived protein inhibits the development of food-allergic reactions in mice. Clin Exp Allergy 2003; 33(11):1595–602.
[81] Lee SY, Huang CK, Zhang TF, et al. Oral administration of IL-12 suppresses anaphylactic reactions in a murine model of peanut hypersensitivity. Clin Immunol 2001;101(2): 220–8.
[82] Garrett JK, Jameson SC, Thomson B, et al. Anti-interleukin-5 (mepolizumab) therapy for hypereosinophilic syndromes. J Allergy Clin Immunol 2004;113(1):115–9.

ELSEVIER
SAUNDERS

Immunol Allergy Clin N Am
27 (2007) 129–139

IMMUNOLOGY
AND ALLERGY
CLINICS
OF NORTH AMERICA

A Rice-Based Edible Vaccine Expressing Multiple T-Cell Epitopes to Induce Oral Tolerance and Inhibit Allergy

Fumio Takaiwa, PhD

Transgenic Crop Research and Development Center, National Institute of Agrobiological Sciences, Kannondai 2-1-2, Tsukuba, Ibaraki 305-8602, Japan

Japanese cedar (*Cryptomeria japonica*) pollinosis is the predominant seasonal allergic disease in Japan, with rhinitis and conjunctivitis as clinical symptoms from February to April each year. Epidemiologic studies indicate that approximately 20% of the Japanese population is afflicted with this allergic disease [1]. Furthermore, more than half of the general population has specific circulating IgE for cedar pollen allergens. The number of patients who have *Cryptomeria* pollinosis and the economic costs associated with this disease are expected to increase steadily, resulting in a strong social demand for the development of a reliable and effective way to control it.

In general, allergen avoidance, pharmacotherapy, and immunotherapy are the three principle treatments for allergic diseases [2]. The main strategy for treating allergic diseases is based on pharmacologic therapy. Many therapeutic medicines against allergic diseases have been developed that block the release of chemical mediators of the inflammatory response, such as histamine, leukotrienes, and prostaglandins. Intranasal corticosteroids and antihistamines have been used to ameliorate allergy symptoms in the mucous membranes, where the inflammatory response is propagated.

However, treatment using these pharmacologic therapies reduces clinical symptoms but does not provide a cure for allergic diseases, and several contraindications and side effects are associated with these drugs. Therefore, a treatment that addresses the immunologic causes of allergic disease would be a significant boon to society. Allergen-specific immunotherapy is a cornerstone in the management of allergic diseases and is the only treatment that

This work was supported by research grants "Research for the utilization and industrialization of agricultural biotechnology" and "Functional analysis of genes relevant to agriculturally important traits in rice genome" from the Ministry of Agriculture, Forestry and Fisheries of Japan.

E-mail address: takaiwa@nias.affrc.go.jp

doi:10.1016/j.iac.2006.11.001 *immunology.theclinics.com*

can interfere with the basic pathophysiologic mechanisms of allergic disease [3].

Systemic immunization with protein extracts from several pollen sources has been shown to be an effective therapeutic treatment [4]. The clinical effects obtained through allergen-specific immunotherapy are the result of a decrease in allergen-specific IgE, an increase in blocking IgG, an increase in type 1 T-helper (Th1) cytokines, and a reduction in allergen-specific T-cell responsiveness. However, in conventional allergen-specific immunotherapy, repeated hypodermic administration with increasing doses of natural allergen extracts over the course of up to 3 years is required for effective and long-term results. Missing or delaying a treatment requires a regression in dose, thus extending the required treatment period. Because this regimen can be difficult to maintain, many patients drop out of treatment. This regimen also has a risk for severe adverse events, such as anaphylactic shock and pain from inflammation at the injection site, because intact allergens are subcutaneously administrated. Because of the risks involved, systemic administration of allergens must be performed in a clinical setting. Therefore, development of a safe, effective, and convenient allergen-specific immunotherapy is needed. An edible vaccine (oral treatment) could be a desirable alternative to current treatments.

To avoid IgE-mediated complications and decrease the length of treatment, oral peptide immunotherapy using T-cell epitopes derived from allergens has been applied in mice as an animal model. This alternative therapy is possible because the specific T-cell activity responsible for the antigen-specific immune reaction can be modulated through not only subcutaneous and intradermal injection but also oral administration of specific T-cell epitopes [5,6].

This article reviews progress in the area of oral administration of rice plants containing T-cell epitopes derived from Japanese cedar pollen allergens. In an important series of proof-of-concept experiments, transgenic rice seeds were fed to mice to induce oral immune tolerance before challenging with pollen allergens. This study showed a significant reduction of allergy symptoms in the test mice and a decrease in allergen-specific IgE and histamine levels from suppression of the specific T-cell reaction. Transgenic rice seed that accumulates allergen-specific T-cell epitopes can thus be expected to act as a new type of tolerogen for suppressing allergen-specific $CD4^+$ T-cell reactivity and to provide a new approach for the immunotherapy of allergic diseases. Furthermore, advantages of rice seed–based peptide vaccines include low cost of production, simple administration, negligible risk for contamination with human or animal pathogens, and low risk for negative immune reactions.

Characterization of Japanese cedar pollen allergen proteins and their T-cell epitope peptides

Two major allergens of Japanese cedar pollen, Cry j 1 and Cry j 2, have been isolated and characterized. More than 90% of patients who have

Japanese cedar pollinosis had IgE specific to both allergens [7]. Cry j 1 is a basic glycoprotein pectate lyase with an apparent molecular weight of 41 to 45 kd and isoelectric point (pI) of 8.9 to 9.2 [8]. Cry j 2 is also a basic protein with polygalacturonate activity and a molecular weight of 37 kd and pI of 8.6 to 8.8 [9]. Both proteins are specifically localized in the cell walls of papilla and amyloplasts in cedar pollen. The nucleotide sequences of the Cry j 1 [8,10] and Cry j 2 cDNAs [9,11] have been determined and their amino acid sequences have been deduced from their nucleotide sequences. T-cell determinants in Cry j 1 and Cry j 2 have been characterized by measuring the proliferative responses of peripheral blood monoclonuclear cells (PMBC) from patients who have Japanese cedar pollinosis to overlapping peptide fragments covering the entire length of the allergen peptides. Optimized T-cell epitopes without IgE binding were determined by two Japanese research groups [12,13]. Three amino acid sequences from Cry j1 (p212–224, p235–247, and p312–330) and four amino acid sequences from Cry j 2 (p77–89, p96–107, p192–204, and p356–367) were identified as being of a suitable size for major human T-cell epitopes using a primary proliferative response assay of freshly isolated PBMC [12]. Two amino acid sequences from Cry j 1 (p108–120, p211–225) and three amino acid sequences from Cry j 2 (p66–80, p182–200, p344–355) were determined by other groups [13]. Both groups identified four of the five T-cell epitopes as potential tolerogens.

T-cell epitopes derived from allergens, which are recognized by specific T cells, vary because they have different haplotypes of the human leukocyte antigen (HLA) II class molecules. This variation is a serious problem for the development of peptide immunotherapy that takes advantage of T-cell epitope peptides. To overcome this problem, artificial hybrid epitope peptides composed of several T-cell epitopes derived from the same allergen or a few allergens were created. Several major T-cell epitopes were chosen to be included in the design of an artificial hybrid polypeptide in which these five or seven candidate T-cell epitopes, derived from different allergen molecules, were linked together [13,14]. Hybrid T-cell epitope peptides have several benefits when used as immunotherapeutic tolerogens [14]. These peptides exhibit little IgE binding activity because B-cell epitopes are eliminated, and the novel combinations result in conformational changes. For example, the hybrid seven-linked epitope (7Crp epitope) showed no binding to specific IgE in the serum of 48 patients who had Japanese cedar pollinosis symptoms [14]. The 7Crp peptide induced T-cell proliferation with an average concentration 100-fold lower than a mixture of the T-cell epitopes. Immunogenicity comparable to the response to native Cry j 1 and Cry j 2 allergens is retained even by the form of the hybrid peptide composed of several T-cell epitopes. The major T-cell epitopes from Cry j 1 and Cry j 2 were also determined using T cells from mice immunized with these antigens. The T cells of B10.S mice immunized with Cry j 1 were reported to recognize three amino sequences, p111–130, p211–230, and p310–330 [15], whereas the two amino acid sequences (Cry j 1 p277–290 and Cry j 2 p246–258) were identified as major T-cell epitopes in BALB/c mice using overlapping peptides [16]. Cry j 2 p70–83 was identified as a minor T-cell epitope [16].

Oral administration of the immunodominant Cry j 2 p246–258 T-cell epitope peptide in BALB/c mice four times at intervals of 3 or 4 days for 14 days before challenging with Cry j 2 allergen results in suppression of T-cell proliferation, specific IgE, and histamine release by mast cells, indicating that oral feeding of T-cell epitopes can result in immune tolerance [17]. The potential for peptide-based oral immunotherapy was first shown by this experiment. The immunogenicity and tolerogenicity of each T-cell epitope and in the linked epitope peptide were apparently also retained, because oral administration of three linked BALB/c mouse T-cell epitopes inhibited T-cell proliferation against the three T-cell epitopes [16].

Mucosal immune tolerance

Oral tolerance is the most common response of the host to the environment. Development of oral tolerance is an important natural mechanism whereby the host becomes tolerant to ingested food proteins and other antigens. This induction of immune tolerance can be provided by direct mucosal exposure to antigens. Therefore, the development of mucosal tolerance through oral immunization against pollen antigens could be an essential and powerful tool for inhibiting allergic reactions, including IgE-mediated hypersensitivities such as type I allergic disease [18,19].

Oral tolerance in mice occurs after either administration of a single high dose of antigen (10–500 mg) or repeated exposure to lower doses (1–5 mg) [20]. These high- and low-dose tolerances are mediated by separate and distinct mechanisms [20]. Clonal deletion and anergy, which can be elicited by large doses of antigen (high-dose tolerance), are characterized by the absence of antigen-specific T-cell proliferation and decreased interleukin (IL)-2 production, resulting in oral tolerance [20,21]. High-dose oral tolerance–induced deletion can be mediated by high-affinity T-cell receptor (TCR) crosslinking or by inhibitory ligands CD95 through CD95, leading to apoptosis. Anergy occurs when incomplete activation signals are sent through TCR interactions between factors such as CD80 or CD86 on antigen-presenting cells with CD28 on T cells (low-affinity interaction) or when a lack of costimulation molecules occurs during activity. However, low-dose tolerance is mediated by the active suppression of immune responses by T cells [19,20]. It is controlled by regulatory T cells that can be divided into three subsets, such as $CD4^{+}CD25^{+}$ natural regulatory T cells, Th3 cells, and Tr1 cells [19,20]. $CD4^{+}CD25^{+}$ regulatory T cells express high levels of cytotoxic T lymphocyte antigen 4 (CTLA4) molecules and the immunosuppressive cytokines IL-10 and transforming growth factor beta (TGF-β). TGF-β–producing Th3 cells have also been implicated in low-dose tolerance [19,20]. Active suppression of the immune responses is therefore achieved through cognate interactions and soluble (IL-10, TGF-β) or cell-surface–associated suppressive cytokines.

Rice seed–based edible vaccines as an effective treatment for cedar pollen allergies

Allergen-specific immunotherapy using intact native allergens has been used successfully to treat allergic diseases, but this type of therapy has been associated with an increased risk for systemic anaphylaxis mediated by allergen-specific IgE. To avoid these side effects, peptide immunotherapy using dominant T-cell epitopes was proposed as a treatment alternative [21,22]. Peptide immunotherapy has been mainly performed through systemic injection, intranasal application, or oral administration in animal models. These treatments result in a reduction in allergen-specific T-cell proliferation and IgE levels, and in changes in the pattern of cytokine release by Th2 cells. Shifts in the immunologic balance from allergen-specific Th2 to Th1 or Th0 cytokine, or down-regulation of the cytokine response released from Th1 and Th2 cells have been observed after treatment with a peptide vaccine [23].

As a new immunotherapy based on the principle of peptide immunotherapy, rice seeds that accumulate major T-cell epitopes derived from pollen allergens were used as a vehicle to deliver mucosal tolerogens. To confirm the oral tolerogenic efficacy of a rice seed–based edible vaccine, transgenic rice seed containing only the BALB/c mice major T-cell epitope peptides Cry j 1 p277–290 and Cry j 2 p246–59 was created [24]. Because these short T-cell epitopes could not be expressed directly, they were introduced into variable regions of the soybean seed storage protein glycinin (A1aB1b) as a fusion protein (Fig. 1). The epitopes are thus expressed as part of a stable storage protein. After the endosperm-specific 2.3-kb glutelin *GluB-1* promoter and the 0.6Kb *GluB-1* terminator were ligated to this fusion protein gene, the entire expression vector was transferred into the rice genome through *Agrobacterium*-mediated transformation. The modified glycinin-containing major mouse T-cell epitopes were thus specifically expressed in the endosperm of transgenic rice seeds under the control of the rice major seed storage protein glutelin *GluB-1* promoter [24]. The modified glycinin accumulated at a level of 7 μg per grain (0.5% of total seed protein) in mature rice seeds. When 10 transgenic rice seeds (70 μg modified glycinin; 2 μg total epitope dose) were fed daily to mice for 4 weeks, the mice had far less of an immune reaction to pollen in a systemic challenge than mice fed nontransgenic rice controls, indicating that the rice seed–based vaccine induced oral immune tolerance. Treated mice showed not only significant reductions in the specific $CD^{+}4$ T-cell proliferative reaction but also reduced allergen-specific IgE and IgG levels and production of IL-4, IL-5, and IL-13 associated with allergen-specific Th2 cells; histamine release from mast cells was also inhibited by feeding with the transgenic rice seeds [24]. The clinical symptoms of allergy

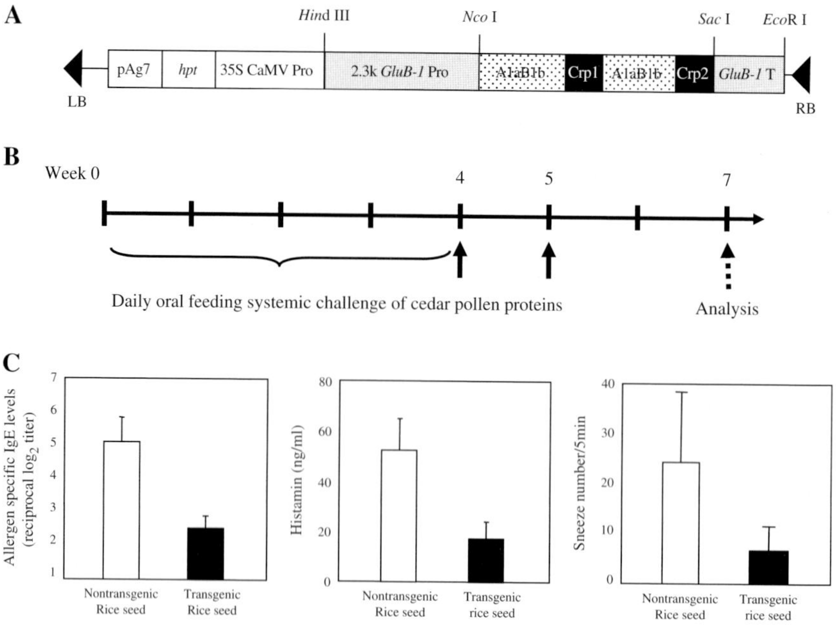

Fig. 1. Oral immune suppression induced by feeding transgenic rice seeds accumulating A1aB1b containing major mouse T-cell epitopes derived from Cry j 1 and Cry j 2 allergens. (*A*) Schematic presentation of the binary vector used for expression of the modified A1aB1b in transgenic rice seed. (*B*) Feeding schedule and challenge with cedar pollen allergens. (*C*) Inhibition of allergen-specific serum IgE, serum histamine and the number of sneezes by oral administration of transgenic rice seeds compared with nontransgenic rice seeds. 35S CaMV Pro, cauliflower mosaic virus 35S promoter; *GluB-1* Pro, rice glutelin *GluB-1* promoter; *hpt*, hygromycin phosphotransferase gene; LB, left border; pAg7, agropine synthase polyadenylation signal sequence; RB, right border.

(sneezing) were also suppressed when assayed in an experimental sneezing mouse model [24]. These results showed that oral immune tolerance was induced by administering transgenic rice seeds containing the major T-cell epitopes.

A human version of the transgenic rice seed–based edible vaccine against Japanese cedar pollinosis was generated based on the feasibility of an oral peptide immunotherapy strategy against pollen allergy using rice seed–based vaccines in mice. An artificial hybrid peptide *7Crp* gene encoding a 96 amino acid protein of seven-linked human dominant T-cell epitope peptides derived from Cry j 1 and Cry j 2 allergens was synthesized using codons optimized for expression in rice seed [25]. To enhance accumulation of the 7Crp peptide, nucleotide sequences for the *N*-terminal GluB-1 signal peptide and *C*-terminal KDER ER retention signal were ligated to *7Crp*. The 7Crp peptide was specifically accumulated in mature seeds at a maximum level of approximately 60 μg per grain (4% of total seed protein) under the control of the

2.3-kb glutelin *GluB-1* promoter in transgenic rice plants generated by *Agrobacterium*-mediated transformation (Fig. 2). Like glutelin, the 7Crp peptide is coordinately synthesized during seed maturation, and is specifically accumulated in the endosperm, whereas leaf, stem, and embryo tissues have no signal [25]. Intracellular localization was examined using immunoelectron microscopy. 7Crp was predominantly deposited in protein bodies in the rice endosperm despite the attachment of the KDEL ER retention signal [25].

Transgenic rice seeds (560 μg total dose of 7Crp) were administered orally to B10.S mice for 32 days and then the mice were nasally challenged with intact Cry j 1 allergen. B10.S mice recognize only one epitope (Cry j 1 p211–225), but the T-cell proliferative responses and serum IgE levels against Cry j 1 were depressed compared with control mice fed nontransgenic rice seeds, thus indicating the potential usefulness of the transgenic 7Crp seeds for controlling pollen allergy in humans [25]. T-cell proliferative activity (ie, immunogenicity) is retained even after boiling 7Crp rice for 20 minutes at 100°C or autoclaving for 20 minutes, indicating that oral immune tolerance would be effective with steamed or cooked rice. This observation suggests that rice seed–based edible vaccine could be provided in a form familiar to Japanese consumers, and thus may be a practical

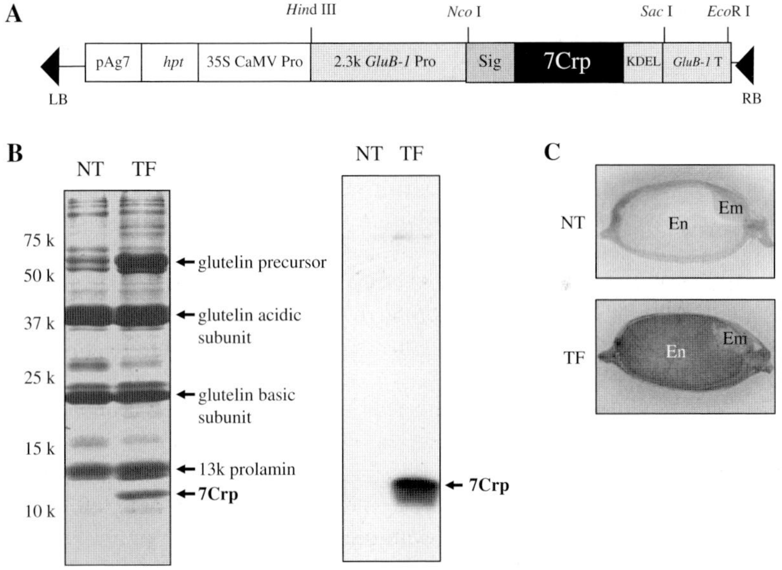

Fig. 2. Expression of 7Crp epitope peptide in transgenic rice seed. (*A*) Schematic of the construct used for expression of 7Crp in transgenic rice seed. (*B*) Accumulation of 7Crp in transgenic rice seed. Coomassie brilliant blue–stained SDS-PAGE of total proteins extracted from the seeds of nontransgenic (NT) and transgenic (TF) rice. Expression was confirmed by Western blotting using specific anti-7Crp serum. (*C*) In situ immunolocalization of 7Crp in transgenic seed. En, endosperm; Em, embryo.

treatment for cedar pollinosis. An effective human dose of 7Crp for inducing oral tolerance to Japanese cedar pollen was extrapolated from the effective dose (2 μg) for mice and the mean relative body weights of mice (30 g) and humans (60 kg). The consumption of approximately 12 g of 7Crp rice (at approximately 50 μg per 20 mg of grain) per day should be sufficient. Japanese citizens eat approximately 100 g of rice per day as a staple food, and therefore 7Crp seed can be used to supplement the daily diet through mixing with normal rice.

The food safety of 7Crp seeds, or of any subsequently developed rice seeds containing immunoactive constituents, must be carefully examined before use. Regulatory standards based on substantial equivalence have been used to determine the food safety of transgenic crops. With this method, a comparative assessment of the toxicology and nutrient composition is made between the newly developed transgenic food and a conventional counterpart. When several macro- and micronutrients were compared between the cognate parental nontransgenic and transgenic 7Crp seeds, the amino acid, lipid, and mineral compositions were essentially identical.

Rice is a new vehicle for production and delivery of edible vaccines

Artificial T-cell epitope peptides used as tolerogens have been produced in recombinant bacteria or yeasts and then extracted and purified for peptide immunotherapy. This production must be performed at a facility that has pharmacologic technology, and the purification process is very costly. In contrast, peptide vaccines produced in the edible parts of crops makes large-scale production efficient, accessible, and responsive to demand, because direct delivery is achievable without the need for purification or partition into effective doses. These advantages of plant-based production offer a simpler and cheaper method of vaccine mass production.

Pharmaceutical proteins produced in transgenic plants generally have not been targeted to specific tissues, but have been expressed broadly in the vegetative tissues such as leaves, roots, fruits, and tubers or seeds using CaMV 35S or maize ubiquitin-1 constitutive promoters. Expression and accumulation of these proteins is in most cases limited to less than 1% of total protein [26,27]. If edible vaccines are to be clinically effective, sufficient levels of the active peptides must be produced and accumulated in the food-use tissues. Low levels of expression can be overcome by increasing promoter activity or by changing the target tissue, subcellular location, plant species, genetic background, codon use of the transgene, post-translational signal sequences, or other factors [28]. Transgene products expressed in leaves, tubers, and roots are not highly accumulated irrespective of high levels of mRNA transcripts.

Seed is the ideal plant production site because it is a natural storage organ that accumulates storage proteins, starch, and lipids, offering ample storage space for foreign recombinant proteins [29]. Seed-specific promoters with high activity have been reported in rice, maize, common bean, and wheat [29], and compartment-specific promoters were recently developed in rice [30]. The *β-glucuronidase* reporter gene can be highly expressed in the rice aleurone, subaleurone, and inner starchy endosperm under the control of the 10-kd prolamin, glutelin *GluB* subfamily, and 26-kd globulin promoters, respectively [30]. The tissues and subcellular compartments suitable for accumulation may differ on a case-by-case basis depending on the tolerogen.

As a production system, rice seed has several advantages over other cereal crops, including easier storage and processing, greater biomass (yield per unit area), and the fact that it is essentially self-crossing and can be grown at a lower cost to the producer. In addition, a transformation system has been established and the whole genome has been sequenced. The 7Crp epitope peptide is stably accumulated only in the seed endosperm tissue of transgenic rice, even though high transcript levels were observed in seed embryos, leaves, stems, and roots. Accumulation levels can also be increased by changing the genetic background of a host. For example, a low storage protein mutant could provide additional storage capacity for introduced gene products [31,32]. Two- to threefold differences have been reported in accumulation levels among hosts with different genetic backgrounds. Furthermore, recombinant proteins expressed in seed are stable for more than a year even if stored at room temperature. The combination of peptide stability without refrigeration, high accumulation levels, and targeting of the product to specific edible tissues indicates that seed is by far the best organ to serve as a natural bioreactor.

Vaccine proteins accumulated in the seed are more resistant than conventional purified protein vaccines to enzymatic digestion in the gastrointestinal tract. Therefore, much smaller amounts of edible vaccine can delivered as a seed storage protein and still effectively induce oral tolerance. To be effective, antigens must be delivered through M cells in Peyer's patches and intestinal epithelial cells in gut-associated lymphoid tissue (GALT) to induce immune tolerance. Efficacy at lower concentrations may be caused by the concentration of antigens through packaging in the plant cell wall and further concentrated by compartmentalization in specialized protein body organelles.

Another approach may include enhancing the efficacy of delivery to the mucosal immune system using mucosal adjuvants [20,33]. The cholera toxin B-subunit (CTB) is a candidate adjuvant because it has been implicated in the induction of specific mucosal immune responses. Expression of T-cell epitopes as a fusion protein with CTB may induce immune tolerance at a much smaller concentration because of binding of CTB to M cells through the polysaccharide GM-1 ganglioside as CTB receptor on the intestinal epithelium. This process would result in site-specific delivery and presentation of the active peptide to the GALT. CTB may also increase the molar concentration of the antigen through pentamerization, resulting in a further increase in antigen concentration at the GALT [33].

Bringing a rice seed–based edible vaccine to market

Many hurdles must be cleared before transgenic rice seed edible vaccines can be brought to market. Several ecologic risks associated with transgene escape during cultivation and transport remain unresolved with genetically altered crops in general [34]. Cross-contamination of seeds during the distribution process (product contamination) and out-crossing with neighboring nontransgenic rice (genetic hybridization) are also unresolved concerns. These risks, however, can be controlled through regulatory measures. Biopharmaceutical plants may need to be grown in a contained environment, with either physical or geographic isolation. An easily recognizable marker may be introduced to discriminate between the edible vaccine rice and normal nontransgenic rice, such as anthocyanins or other natural plant pigments, which would essentially color-code the engineered seeds. On the other hand, incorporating selectable marker genes that confer resistance to antibiotics would need to be eliminated during commercialization. Marker-free transgenic rice plants harboring the 7Crp gene have already been established using only the multi-auto-transformation (MAT) vector system.

References

[1] Kaneko Y, Motohashi Y, Nakamura H, et al. Increasing prevalence of Japanese cedar pollinosis: a meta-regression analysis. Int Arch Allergy Immunol 2005;136:365–71.

[2] Walker SM, Varney VA, Gaga M, et al. Grass pollen immunotherapy: efficacy and safety during a 4-year follow-up study. Allergy 1995;50:405–13.

[3] Frew AJ. Immunotherapy of allergic disease. J Allergy Clin Immunol 2003;111:S712–9.

[4] Bousquet J, Van Cauwenberge P, editors. Allergic rhinitis and its impact on asthma. J Allergy Clin Immunol 2001;108(Suppl 5): S240–5.

[5] Hoyne DF, Kristensen NM, Yssel H, et al. Peptide modulation of allergen-specific immne responses. Curr Opin Immunol 1995;7:757–61.

[6] Garside P, Mowat AM. Oral tolerance. Semin Immunol 2001;13:177–85.

[7] Hashimoto M, Nigi H, Sakaguchi M, et al. Sensitivity to two major allergens (Cry j I and Cry j II) in patients with Japanese cedar (*Cryptomeria japonica*) pollinosis. Clin Exp Allergy 1995;25:848–52.

[8] Yasueda H, Yui Y, Shimizu T, et al. Isolation and partial characterization of the major allergen from Japanese cedar (*Cryptomeria japonica*) pollen. J Allergy Clin Immunol 1983;71: 77–86.

[9] Sone T, Komiyama N, Shimizu K, et al. Cloning and sequencing of cDNA coding for Cry j 1, a major allergen of Japanese cedar pollen. Biochem Biophys Res Commun 1994;199:619–25.

[10] Sakaguchi M, Inouye S, Taniai M, et al. Identification of the second major allergen of Japanese cedar pollen. Allergy 1990;45:309–12.

[11] Namba M, Kurose M, Torigoe K, et al. Molecular cloning of the second major allergen, Cry j II, from Japanese cedar pollen. FEBS Lett 1994;353:124–8.

[12] Saito S, Hirahara K, Kawaguchi J, et al. Identification of T cell determinants in Cry j 1 and Cry j 2 of size suitable for peptide immunotherapy against Japanese cedar pollinosis. Ann Rep Sankyo Res Lab 2000;52:49–58.
[13] Sone T, Komiyama N, Shimizu K, et al. T cell epitopes in Japanese cedar (Cryptomeria japonica) pollen allergens: choice of major T cell epitopes in Cry j1 and Cryj2 toward design of the peptide-based immunotherapeutics for management of Japanese cedar pollinosis. J Immunol 1998;161:448–57.
[14] Hirahara K, Tatsuta T, Takatori T, et al. Preclinical evaluation of an immunotherapeutic peptide comprising 7 T-cell determinants of Cry j1 and Cry j2, the major Japanese cedar pollen allergens. J Allergy Clin Immunol 2001;108:94–100.
[15] Ohno N, Sakaguchi M, Inouye S. et al. Common antigenicity between Japanese cedar (Cryptomeria japonica) pollen and Japanese cypress (Chamaecyparis obtusa) pollen, II. Determination of the cross-reacting T-cell epitope of Cry j 1 and Cha o1 in mice. Immunology 2000; 99:630–4.
[16] Yoshitomi T, Hirahara K, Kawaguchi J, et al. Three T-cell determinants of Cry j1 and Cry j2, the major Japanese cedar pollen antigens, retain their immunogenicity and tolerogenicity in a linked peptide. Immunology 2002;107:517–22.
[17] Hirahara K, Saito S, Serizawa N, et al. Oral administration of a dominant T-cell determinant peptide inhibits allergen-specific TH1 and TH2 cell response in Cry j2-primed mice. J Allergy Clin Immunol 1998;102:961–7.
[18] Strobel S. Oral tolerance, systemic immunoregulation, and autoimmunity. Ann N Y Acad Sci 2002;958:45–58.
[19] Faria AC, Weiner HL. Oral tolerance. Immunol Rev 2005;206:232–59.
[20] Mayer L, Shao L. Therapeutic potential of oral tolerance. Nat Rev Immunol 2004;4:407–19.
[21] Wallner BP, Gefter ML. Peptide therapy for treatment of allergic diseases. Clin Immunol Immunopathol 1996;80:105–9.
[22] Haselden BM, Kay AB, Larche M. Peptide-mediated immune responses in specific immunotherapy. Int Arch Allergy Immunol 2000;122:229–37.
[23] Larche M, Wraith DC. Peptide-based therapeutic vaccines for allergic and autoimmune diseases. Nat Med 2005;11:569–76.
[24] Takagi H, Hiroi T, Yang L, et al. A rice-based edible vaccine expressing multiple epitopes induces oral tolerance for inhibition of Th2-mediated IgE responses. Proc Natl Acad Sci U S A 2005;102:17525–30.
[25] Takagi H, Saito S, Yang L, et al. Oral immunotherapy against a pollen allergy using a seed-based peptide vaccine. Plant Biotechnol J 2005;3:521–33.
[26] Daniell H, Streatfield SJ, Wycoff K. Medical molecular farming: production of antibodies, biopharmaceuticals and edible vaccines in plants. Trends Plant Sci 2001;6:219–26.
[27] Stoger E, Sack M, Perrin Y, et al. Practical considerations for pharmaceutical antibody production in different systems. Mol Breed 2002;9:149–58.
[28] Sala F, Rigano MM, Barbante A, et al. Vaccine antigen production in transgenic plants: strategies, gene constructs and perspectives. Vaccine 2003;21:803–8.
[29] Stoger E, Ma JKC, Fischer R, et al. Sowing the seeds of success: pharmaceutical proteins from plants. Curr Opin Biotechnol 2005;16:167–73.
[30] Qu LQ, Takaiwa F. Tissue specific expression and quantitative potential evaluate of seed storage component gene promoters in transgenic rice. Plant Biotechnol J 2004;2:113–25.
[31] Tada Y, Utsumi S, Takaiwa F. Foreign gene products can be enhanced by introduction into low storage protein mutants. Plant Biotechnol J 2003;1:411–22.
[32] Twyman RM, Stoger E, Schillberg S, et al. Molecular farming in plants: host systems and expression technology. Trends Biotechnol 2003;21:570–8.
[33] Holmgren J, Czerkinsky C. Mucosal immunity and vaccines. Nat Med 2005;11:S45–53.
[34] Kirk DD, McIntosh K, Walmsley AM, et al. Risk analysis for plan-made vaccines. Transgenic Res 2005;14:449–62.

ELSEVIER
SAUNDERS

Immunol Allergy Clin N Am
27 (2007) 141–144

IMMUNOLOGY
AND ALLERGY
CLINICS
OF NORTH AMERICA

Index

Note: Page numbers of article titles are in **bold face** type.

doi:10.1016/S0889-8561(07)00014-8